Practical Issues in Geriatrics

Series Editor
Stefania Maggi
Aging Branch
CNR-Neuroscience Institute
Padua
Italy

This practically oriented series presents state of the art knowledge on the principal diseases encountered in older persons and addresses all aspects of management, including current multidisciplinary diagnostic and therapeutic approaches. It is intended as an educational tool that will enhance the everyday clinical practice of both young geriatricians and residents and also assist other specialists who deal with aged patients. Each volume is designed to provide comprehensive information on the topic that it covers, and whenever appropriate the text is complemented by additional material of high educational and practical value, including informative video-clips, standardized diagnostic flow charts and descriptive clinical cases. Practical Issues in Geriatrics will be of value to the scientific and professional community worldwide, improving understanding of the many clinical and social issues in Geriatrics and assisting in the delivery of optimal clinical care.

More information about this series at http://www.springer.com/series/15090

Jean-Pierre Michel
Editor

Prevention of Chronic Diseases and Age-Related Disability

Springer

Editor
Jean-Pierre Michel
Geneva University
Geneva
Switzerland

French National Academy of Medicine
Paris
France

ISSN 2509-6060 ISSN 2509-6079 (electronic)
Practical Issues in Geriatrics
ISBN 978-3-030-07209-4 ISBN 978-3-319-96529-1 (eBook)
https://doi.org/10.1007/978-3-319-96529-1

This Springer imprint is published by the registered company Springer Nature Switzerland AG
The registered company address is: Gewerbestrasse 11, 6330 Cham, Switzerland

Preface

The Future of Ageing

Today, aged 40 years, you are enjoying life, your family and friends, in nice surroundings. You are far from thinking that two of your three children will experience great change and live to be centenarians. Longevity is constantly increasing, but you probably don't imagine that when your children are in their thirties, you will be one of two billion people aged over 60 in the world and at risk of suffering from at least one age-related disability.

Ageing is a fantastic opportunity, linked to outstanding progress, notably a decrease in infant mortality, improved hygiene, easier access to food, vaccination and a safer living environment, mainly related to improved socio-economic conditions in many countries in the world. However, we should not forget that there is a clear relationship between the gross domestic product (GDP) of a country and the life expectancy at birth in that country, which explains why in Chad or the Central African Republic, for example, life expectancy at birth is still around 50, whereas in Monaco, life expectancy at birth is now 89 years.

How can we explain such differences, not only in longevity, but also in functional ability and indeed wellness in old age? The explanations are not all that simple, as ageing is a life course process, from conception to the last days of life.

If, during your infancy and adolescence, you are lucky enough to grow up in a medium- or high-resource country, and you are well nourished, physically active and receive a good education, then you will have a greater likelihood of starting adulthood in excellent conditions: proud of your strength, knowledge, skills and multiple competences, and likely also with complete functional and financial autonomy. Unfortunately, the majority of young adults do not have the advantage of such outstanding and advantageous conditions.

After this fundamental period of growth, every adult will have to work increasingly harder, obliging them to limit their physical exercise or become sedentary, while in parallel, they may not give sufficient priority to buccal and dental hygiene (see Chap. 4) and their daily diet and weight (see Chap. 5), and all too often, they acquire unfavourable life habits or behaviours such as smoking (see Chap. 9).

Whatever the conditions of adulthood, be they optimal or not, advancing age will induce insidious changes that occur silently, such as unbalanced diet (Chap. 5), a gradual decrease in skeletal muscles mass, as well as in strength and function (Chap. 6), and a reduction in physiological reserves, signalling the pre-frailty stage (Chap. 7). These changes may also include a slight reduction in walking speed and balance disorders (Chap. 14), while the bones start to become fragile (Chap. 11) and the joints painful (Chap. 12). The convergence of these multiple conditions will lead (perhaps only decades later) to falls and their multiple consequences (Chap. 14). In parallel, depending on your level of education, job complexity and intellectual stimulation, your brain's connectivity network will modulate both cognitive ability and reserve—possibility in a positive way, but maybe negatively (Chap. 13).

This period at midlife, during which we are exposed to major but hidden problems, is very often completely neglected. Currently, it is well established that this period of life is essential to maintaining, or better still, to increasing physical, mental and cognitive abilities, all of which are key factors in determining the future of the ageing process.

Midlife is crucial, because it includes all the personal advantages and risk factors linked to performance within one's own life surroundings (Chap. 17). The various chapters of this book will address these issues individually and will underline how intervention at the midlife period can positively modify the health/functioning trajectory. A growing number of randomized controlled interventions on midlife risk factors are clearly demonstrating the effectiveness of simple actions, such as changing life habits or behaviours, exercising regularly, choosing a better diet as well as controlling targeted and apparently banal risks, with a view to completely changing the ageing process.

This book, mainly inspired by the 2015 World Health Organization definition of "healthy ageing" (Chaps. 17, 18 and 20), perfectly focuses on our personal ability to function well. This is a revolutionary idea, since the classical concept of disease is now dominated by the functional theory of "daily functioning", enabling the emergence of integrated care (Chap. 19), which will enable us to continue doing those "things that are important for each of us", right up until the last part of our own life.

This theory, which is not yet routinely accepted by numerous physicians and organ specialists, needs to be promoted, to engage healthcare professionals to consider not only a disease, but rather the person's whole life trajectory and its consequences for daily life, including wellness. This book aims to convince healthcare professionals that, whatever your gender and socio-economic status (Chap. 18), midlife health promotion and specific targeted preventive measures are essential. For example, one might cite such interventions as adult vaccination (Chap. 15), particularly for those with diabetes (Chap. 7), asthma or respiratory insufficiency (Chap. 8). General practitioners and organ specialists who try their best to control blood pressure often forget the functional consequences of their outstanding interventions, which save large numbers of lives. For example, the progress in cardiopulmonary resuscitation and treatment of acute kidney failure has been outstanding, yet the survivors of such interventions too often become "ill survivors", who will go on to develop heart failure, chronic renal insufficiency and the inevitable daily disability these conditions entail (Chap. 7). Similarly, oncologists are increasingly focusing on cancer prevention and high-tech long-term management of survivors to personalize their exams and complementary treatments (Chap. 10).

Fortunately, numerous other pathologies are easier to control or prevent at midlife. For instance, undergoing sight and hearing assessment at midlife is fundamental, as sensory dysfunctions are particularly disabling yet easy to avoid (Chap. 14). It is also well known that the combination of overweight, hypertension and hypercholesterolemia at midlife is associated with a sixfold increase in the risk of becoming demented a few decades later (Chap. 13). Why not simply tell people at risk what will happen if they don't completely change their life habits? It is also well established that daily intake of virgin olive oil or nuts decreases adverse cardiovascular events and protects against cognitive decline (Chap. 13). Mouth hygiene and dental care at midlife will not only make it possible to avoid respiratory infection or increasing incidental myocardial infarction, but will help to maintain taste and indeed better nutrient intake throughout life (Chap. 5).

Moreover, our world will continue to see extraordinary progress in high technology, which will greatly benefit the youngest and midlife adults. The possibility of e-health self-assessment, with personalized life advice, and careful follow-up, will totally change the management of the life course in the coming years. It will enable ageing in the home, and ensure security, care safety, independence and communication, while providing improved well-being and avoiding frequent and costly institutionalization.

By acting positively all along your life course, you will become the main actor of your ageing process, which depends on thousands of genes whose expression can be modified by your culture, religion, life habits and behaviours, physical activity and diet. This means that we will be able to age, free of any disability and enjoying well-being up to very old age, surrounded by a growing number of family members and friends in a technologically advanced society that we will have to master as soon as possible, whatever our age.

The comprehensive range of issues addressed in this book will provide the reader with a better understanding of the idea that the adult gap in preventive care is at the origin of preventable, age-related disability. The importance of this concept is not only in improving daily functioning but also in enhancing overall wellness. Moreover, it will be cost-effective for all societies who currently fear that ageing will become an immeasurable burden within a few decades.

It is never too late to become an active player in your own ageing process.

Geneva, Switzerland
Paris, France

Jean-Pierre Michel

Contents

1 A Life Course Approach to Healthy Ageing

Diana Kuh

Key Messages

- A life course epidemiological approach to ageing studies how different capacities change across life for different populations, and whether there are periods of rapid change or transitions where exposures may have particularly long-term consequences for later life health.
- Those who experience socioeconomic disadvantage, or have poorer childhood growth or cognitive development, are less likely to survive to old age, have lower intrinsic capacity and a greater risk of decline.
- A lower level or an accelerated decline in physical and mental capacities by midlife is also associated with lower survival chances and a greater risk of disability and chronic disease.
- Promotion of healthy ageing needs to start early and continue across life.
- Those who take exercise, eat a healthy diet, maintain a normal weight, and do not smoke have a higher level of capacity and a slower rate of decline as they grow older.
- Health professionals need to consider intervening when there is accelerated decline and not necessarily wait until clinical thresholds are reached.

1.1 Introduction

The WHO is promoting a life course approach to healthy ageing [1]. This approach alerts us to: (1) the idea that ageing, the gradual accumulation of molecular and cellular damage, occurs throughout life; (2) the importance of monitoring, investigating,

D. Kuh
MRC National Survey of Health and Development, MRC Unit for Lifelong Health and Ageing at University College London, London, UK
e-mail: d.kuh@ucl.ac.uk

J.-P. Michel (ed.), *Prevention of Chronic Diseases and Age-Related Disability*, Practical Issues in Geriatrics, https://doi.org/10.1007/978-3-319-96529-1_1

and explaining how health is maintained at each life stage, not just in old age; and (3) the opportunities for promoting healthy ageing across life.

The contribution of this opening chapter is to demonstrate the value of the life course epidemiological approach to healthy ageing. Life course epidemiology [2, 3] is part of an interdisciplinary life course perspective on health, development, and ageing that has grown strongly in recent years [4]. Such an approach extends the WHO healthy ageing initiative by developing an understanding of the natural history of the growth, maintenance, and decline in physical and mental (cognitive and emotional) capacities across life, and how social and biological factors in childhood, early and middle adult life act independently or interactively to impair capacity leading to disability and chronic disease in later life. In this chapter, the focus is on the factors affecting physical capacity in early and middle adulthood, and the consequences of midlife capacity for later disability and disease.

From a policy perspective, the life course approach highlights when preventive strategies may be most effective. Early life prevention includes strategies for enhancing physical and mental capacities during growth and development; midlife prevention includes strategies for maintaining capacity for as long as possible after maturity by delaying the onset of decline.

Integral to a life course approach is the investigation of the impact of birth cohort, and lifetime social stratification (including the social relations governing the economic structure, gender, and ethnicity), on healthy ageing and the drivers and consequences of these group differences.

1.2 A Life Course Approach: Conceptual Framework

Life course epidemiology studies lifetime functional trajectories at three different levels: (1) at the individual or multi-system level where the terms physical and cognitive capability are often used to highlight their key roles as hallmarks of ageing and to distinguish them from (2) the functions of underlying body systems on which capability depends [5]. Using WHO terminology, both these levels of function would come under intrinsic capacity, and this chapter will therefore use this term. A life course approach is also being increasingly applied to study (3) changes in function at the molecular and cellular levels, and how these relate to change in intrinsic capacity at the body system or individual levels, a key area of research.

Whether our focus is on the age-related disability and chronic diseases, intrinsic capacity, or the cellular and molecular mechanisms of biological ageing, we need to understand better how they change across life (the life course trajectory) and are affected by the timing and duration of exposure to social and physical environmental factors acting right across life, as well as across generations. Health at any stage of life depends on the ability to respond—to resist, compensate, adapt to, and recover from environmental challenges. These responses may take place over different time scales: homeostasis acting over a short time scale, developmental plasticity across life, and natural selection over generations [6]. Big data—data intensive biology—is providing a better understanding of the mechanisms underlying homeostasis and developmental plasticity; evolutionary theories offer a broad interpretative framework. Life course epidemiology studies how different capacities change across life, whether there are periods of rapid change or transitions where physical and social exposures may have more long-term consequences than at other times, and whether there are differences by birth cohorts, socioeconomic position, gender, or ethnicity. It investigates how childhood factors may affect the development of peak capacity and how child and adult factors maintain this peak, delay the onset, or modify the rate of decline. It recognises that while environmental stimuli are required to develop and maintain capacity, other environmental exposures, often highly socially patterned, have long-term damaging consequences. It seeks to understand how those most resilient to adversities draw on intrinsic or extrinsic characteristics in resisting, recovering, compensating, or adapting to these challenges.

1.3 Assessing Trajectories of Intrinsic Capacity

A life course approach ideally requires cohort studies with long term, preferably lifelong follow-up. The UK is particularly fortunate in having a wealth of such studies; this chapter draws on examples from the MRC National Survey of Health and Development (NSHD) which has followed a nationally representative sample of British men and women since their birth in a week in March 1946, and on whom there is a wealth of data from 0 to 70 years [7]. Empirical evidence linking exposures earlier in life to later capacity and other health outcomes initially came from single cohort studies like NSHD, but where sufficient studies are available, systematic reviews, and meta-analyses have been conducted; these provide stronger evidence on which to base changes in policy and practice. Increasingly, the statistical power of cross cohort studies and large cohort studies is being utilised to provide reliable estimates of the associations between risk and protective factors acting at different ages and these later outcomes.

Physical capacity can be assessed by tests of muscle strength (e.g., grip strength), locomotor function (e.g., walking speed, timed get up and go, chair rising), balance (e.g., one legged stands) and dexterity (e.g., pegboard test) [8, 9]. These tests are commonly used in population studies, can be easily applied to a range of settings, and identify meaningful variation between and within individuals from at least as early as midlife; modification and/or substitution of these tests may be required at earlier ages. Similarly, tools that test the domains of cognitive function (e.g., verbal memory, processing speed, executive function) and those that test cardiovascular, lung, and immune function and other body systems relevant to ageing are readily available [9]. Self-reports of intrinsic capacity and functional ability are also important to capture the lived experience and to design intervention strategies.

Evidence to date shows that lifetime trajectories of physical and cognitive capacity generally show an increase in capacity during growth and development, peaking or plateauing at maturity, with an initial slow rate of decline across adulthood that accelerates later in life [10–13].

1.4 Lifetime Influences on Survival to Old Age

Survival to old age can be seen as a necessary but not sufficient condition for healthy ageing, but still needs to be considered given that even some high-income countries are experiencing worrying trends in mortality and life expectancy [14, 15].

A range of social, psychological, and biomedical factors from early life onwards have been shown to affect the risk of premature adult mortality. For example, in NSHD those who grew up in manual households or had lower childhood cognitive ability had a higher risk of dying prematurely than their peers from non-manual households [16]; similar findings have been replicated in many cohort studies [17, 18]. Of relevance to the focus of this book, lower midlife physical capacity was related to a higher mortality rate in NSHD [19], extending previous studies at older ages [20]. Lower cognitive capacity in early adulthood, also related to higher mortality rates, mediated the associations between early life factors (family background, cognitive ability, and education) and adult mortality [21]. These findings suggest that building capacity in childhood and early adult life will improve later life health and survival chances.

1.5 Early and Midlife Influences on Trajectories of Intrinsic Capacity

In NSHD, aspects of poor physical growth, neurodevelopment (delayed motor development, lower childhood cognitive ability, and poorer adolescent motor co-ordination), and early socioeconomic disadvantage have been related to midlife physical capacity in a series of publications (summarised in [8]). Systematic reviews and meta-analyses have strengthened the evidence [22, 23].

Furthermore, there is growing evidence that these early life factors are associated not just with the level but also the rate of decline in adult physical capacity. In NSHD, higher childhood cognitive ability was associated with a lower chance of being in a group who experienced significant decline in grip strength and chair rise performance in the sixth decade of life [24]. In contrast, early socioeconomic disadvantage was associated with a greater chance of being in this group. Additional assessments of grip strength at age 69 have confirmed that the association between lower childhood cognitive ability and lower grip strength has strengthened with age, whereas the pattern of associations of physical growth and motor development with adult grip strength have remained constant.

In addition, adult socioeconomic disadvantage and poorer cognitive function continue to be associated with a lower level of physical capacity and increased risk of decline. However, a healthy adult lifestyle—taking exercise, eating a healthy diet, maintaining a normal weight and not smoking—was associated with a higher level of capacity and a lower chance of decline in the sixth decade [25]. Maintaining physical activity is particularly important for physical capability when taking all the evidence together [26, 27].

The lifetime determinants of mental (cognitive and emotional) capacity are beyond the scope of this chapter. Many factors across life affect the level of adult cognitive capacity (including several associated with physical capacity), and there have been reports of a decline in age-specific dementia incidence or prevalence in several countries; however, identifying factors where there is strong evidence for preventing individual cognitive decline has been more challenging [28, 29]. This again highlights the importance of enhancing and maintaining mental capacity from early life onwards.

1.5.1 Cardio-Metabolic and Respiratory Function

Optimal functioning of cardio-metabolic and respiratory systems are important aspects of intrinsic capacity, underlying many other aspects of functional change. Here, there is a growing wealth of evidence, sometimes obtained by piecing together multiple longitudinal studies with repeated measures covering different periods of the life course, on the changes (including greater heterogeneity) that occur with age [30], their lifetime determinants, and functional and disease consequences [31, 32].

For example, understanding the natural history of lung function and the development of COPD requires a life course perspective. About 50% of COPD cases are due to accelerated decline of FEV1 in adult life but the other 50% already have low FEV1 in early adulthood [33]. Over 40 years ago, the NSHD was one of the first to show that infant lower respiratory tract illness, overcrowding, air pollution and manual paternal occupation were associated with symptoms of chronic bronchitis in young adulthood [34]. Most recently, this study has shown how those who experience this early disadvantage had particularly low levels of midlife lung function if they took up smoking [35]. It is possible that adolescent smoking when the lungs are still developing prevents their recovery from earlier deficits. Those who smoke also have a faster decline in lung function, as do those who experience more episodes of mucus hypersecretion in early and mid-adulthood [36]. Young adulthood is a sensitive period for lung capacity and is an important time for tailored interventions.

There is a wealth of evidence that poor early growth (e.g., lower birthweight or ponderal index) and socioeconomic disadvantage are early determinants of reduced adult cardiovascular and metabolic function [37, 38]. Early disadvantage is related to adverse changes in adult blood pressure, partly due to the earlier and greater increase in adiposity among those from poorer backgrounds [39]. NSHD and other studies have shown that those who have an accelerated rise in blood pressure during early and mid-adulthood are more likely to have adverse indicators of cardiac structure and function and atherosclerosis subsequently [40–42]. Importantly, these associations apply to rises within the normal range of blood pressure raising the question of whether intervention be based on the change in blood pressure, rather than a clinical threshold.

1.5.2 Common Mechanisms Underlying Intrinsic Capacity

There is a growing interest in understanding and potentially modifying the lifetime trajectories and determinants of common ageing phenotypes that underlie many aspects of intrinsic capacity, decline, and variation between social groups; these include changes in body composition, homeostatic dysregulation, and age-related declines in energy efficiency and in central and peripheral nervous system processes [13]. Similarly, a life course perspective would help further understanding of the molecular and cellular mechanisms that may link the epigenome, metabolome, and microbiome (and other -omics data) to healthy ageing.

It is equally important to maintain research and policy interest in the lifetime socioeconomic pathways that influence intrinsic capacity and functional ability. The role of lifetime body composition, particularly adiposity, on intrinsic capacity can hardly be underestimated, and is a good example of the need to integrate both social and biological approaches, supported by a wealth of evidence (e.g., [43, 44]). Here again, factors from early life affect the chance of maintaining a healthy weight [13, 45]. In NSHD, there are striking differences in fat mass in the seventh decade of life, especially for women, by socioeconomic indicators right across life [46]. Cross cohort studies show how childhood and adult social inequalities in lifetime BMI trajectories have been maintained and the overall upward shift in these trajectories [47–49]. These are important trends to tackle, if we are to ensure an equal chance of healthy ageing for all socioeconomic groups.

1.6 Implications for Policy and Practice of a Life Course Approach to Healthy Ageing

Promotion of healthy ageing needs to start early and continue across life. Enhancing the development of intrinsic capacity during growth and development is essential, supported by strong evidence of critical and sensitive periods in early life, and by moral, ethical, and economic arguments to improve child health and reduce social inequalities. In adult life, there needs to be a greater focus on strategies that maintain capacity, and delay the onset and modify the rate of decline. Evidence is growing that early and mid-adulthood is a time of significant functional change when it may be easier to modify the trajectory than at later ages. Health professionals need to consider intervening when there is accelerated decline, and not necessarily wait until clinical thresholds are reached. We also need to identify ways to promote physiological, psychological, and social resilience to maintain intrinsic capacity and functional ability well into old age and improve the well-being of older people.

Acknowledgements Thanks to Dr. Rachel Cooper, Professor Rebecca Hardy, Professor Marcus Richards, and Professor Yoav Ben-Shlomo for their helpful comments on an earlier draft of this chapter.

References

1. World Health Organization (2015) World report on ageing and health
2. Ben-Shlomo Y, Kuh D (2002) A life course approach to chronic disease epidemiology: conceptual models, empirical challenges and interdisciplinary perspectives. Int J Epidemiol 31(2):285–293
3. Kuh D, Ben-Shlomo Y (2004) A life course approach to chronic disease epidemiology, 2nd edn. Oxford University Press, Oxford
4. Ben-Shlomo Y, Cooper R, Kuh D (2016) The last two decades of life course epidemiology, and its relevance for research on ageing. Int J Epidemiol 45(4):973–988
5. Cooper R, Hardy R, Sayers A, Kuh D (2014) A life course approach to physical capability. In: Kuh D, Cooper R, Hardy R, Richards M, Ben-Shlomo Y (eds) A life course approach to healthy ageing, 1st edn. Oxford University Press, Oxford, pp 16–31
6. Gluckman PD, Hanson MA, Bateson P et al (2009) Towards a new developmental synthesis: adaptive developmental plasticity and human disease. Lancet 373(9675):1654–1657
7. Kuh D, Wong A, Shah I et al (2016) The MRC National Survey of Health and Development reaches age 70: maintaining participation at older ages in a birth cohort study. Eur J Epidemiol 31(11):1135–1147
8. Kuh D, Karunananthan S, Bergman H, Cooper R (2014) A life-course approach to healthy ageing: maintaining physical capability. Proc Nutr Soc 73(2):237–248
9. Lara J, Cooper R, Nissan J et al (2015) A proposed panel of biomarkers of healthy ageing. BMC Med 13:222
10. Dodds RM, Syddall HE, Cooper R et al (2014) Grip strength across the life course: normative data from twelve British studies. PLoS One 9(12):e113637
11. Dodds RM, Syddall HE, Cooper R, Kuh D, Cooper C, Sayer AA (2016) Global variation in grip strength: a systematic review and meta-analysis of normative data. Age Ageing 45(2):209–216
12. Davis D, Bendayan R, Muniz G, Hardy R, Richards M, Kuh D (2017) Decline in search speed and verbal memory over 26 years of midlife in a British birth cohort. Neuroepidemiology 49:121–128
13. Ferrucci L, Cooper R, Shardell M, Simonsick EM, Schrack JA, Kuh D (2016) Age-related change in mobility: perspectives from life course epidemiology and geroscience. J Gerontol A Biol Sci Med Sci 71(9):1184–1194
14. Case A, Deaton A (2015) Rising morbidity and mortality in midlife among white non-Hispanic Americans in the 21st century. Proc Natl Acad Sci U S A 112(49):15078–15083
15. Hiam L, Harrison D, McKee M, Dorling D (2018) Why is life expectancy in England and Wales 'stalling'? J Epidemiol Community Health 72:404–408
16. Kuh D, Shah I, Richards M, Mishra G, Wadsworth M, Hardy R (2009) Do childhood cognitive ability or smoking behaviour explain the influence of lifetime socio-economic conditions on premature adult mortality in a British post war birth cohort? Soc Sci Med 68(9):1565–1573
17. Galobardes B, Lynch JW, Smith GD (2008) Is the association between childhood socioeconomic circumstances and cause-specific mortality established? Update of a systematic review. J Epidemiol Community Health 62(5):387–390
18. Calvin CM, Deary IJ, Fenton C et al (2011) Intelligence in youth and all-cause-mortality: systematic review with meta-analysis. Int J Epidemiol 40(3):626–644
19. Cooper R, Strand BH, Hardy R, Patel KV, Kuh D (2014) Physical capability in mid-life and survival over 13 years of follow-up: British birth cohort study. Br Med J 348:g2219
20. Cooper R, Kuh D, Hardy R (2010) Objectively measured physical capability levels and mortality: systematic review and meta-analysis. Br Med J 341:c4467
21. Davis D, Cooper R, Terrera GM, Hardy R, Richards M, Kuh D (2016) Verbal memory and search speed in early midlife are associated with mortality over 25 years' follow-up, independently of health status and early life factors: a British birth cohort study. Int J Epidemiol 45(4):1216–1225

22. Birnie K, Cooper R, Martin RM et al (2011) Childhood socioeconomic position and objectively measured physical capability levels in adulthood: a systematic review and meta-analysis. PLoS One 6(1):e15564
23. Dodds R, Denison HJ, Ntani G et al (2012) Birth weight and muscle strength: a systematic review and meta-analysis. J Nutr Health Ageing 16(7):609–615
24. Cooper R, Richards M, Kuh D (2017) Childhood cognitive ability and age-related changes in physical capability from midlife: findings from a British Birth Cohort Study. Psychosom Med 79(7):785–791
25. Cooper R, Muniz-Terrera G, Kuh D (2016) Associations of behavioural risk factors and health status with changes in physical capability over 10 years of follow-up: the MRC National Survey of Health and Development. BMJ Open 6(4):e009962
26. World Health Organization (2010) Global recommendations on physical activity for health. WHO, Geneva
27. Anton SD, Woods AJ, Ashizawa T et al (2015) Successful aging: advancing the science of physical independence in older adults. Ageing Res Rev 24(Pt B):304–327
28. Leshner AI, Landis S, Stroud C, Downey A, Committee on Preventing Dementia and Cognitive Impairment (2017) Preventing cognitive decline and dementia. The National Academies Press, Washington, DC
29. Livingston G, Sommerlad A, Orgeta V et al (2017) Dementia prevention, intervention, and care. Lancet 390:2673–2734
30. Wills AK, Lawlor DA, Matthews FE et al (2011) Life course trajectories of systolic blood pressure using longitudinal data from eight UK cohorts. PLoS Med 8(6):e1000440
31. Hardy R, Lawlor DA, Kuh D (2015) A life course approach to cardiovascular aging. Future Cardiol 11(1):101–113
32. Lawlor DA, Hardy R (2014) Vascular and metabolic function across the life course. In: Kuh D, Cooper R, Hardy R, Richards M, Ben-Shlomo Y (eds) A life course approach to healthy ageing, 1st edn. Oxford University Press, Oxford, pp 146–161
33. Lange P, Celli B, Agusti A et al (2015) Lung-function trajectories leading to chronic obstructive pulmonary disease. N Engl J Med 373(2):111–122
34. Colley JRT, Douglas JWB, Reid DD (1973) Respiratory disease in young adults; influence of early childhood lower respiratory tract illness, social class, air pollution, and smoking. Br Med J 3:195–198
35. Allinson JP, Hardy R, Donaldson GC, Shaheen SO, Kuh D, Wedzicha JA (2017) Combined impact of smoking and early life exposures on adult lung function trajectories. Am J Respir Crit Care Med 196:1021–1030
36. Allinson JP, Hardy R, Donaldson GC, Shaheen SO, Kuh D, Wedzicha JA (2016) The presence of chronic mucus hypersecretion across adult life in relation to chronic obstructive pulmonary disease development. Am J Respir Crit Care Med 193(6):662–672
37. Whincup PH, Kaye SJ, Owen CG et al (2008) Birth weight and risk of type 2 diabetes: a systematic review. JAMA 300(24):2886–2897
38. Galobardes B, Smith GD, Lynch JW (2006) Systematic review of the influence of childhood socioeconomic circumstances on risk for cardiovascular disease in adulthood. Ann Epidemiol 16(2):91–104
39. Hardy R, Kuh D, Langenberg C, Wadsworth M (2003) Birthweight, childhood social class, and change in adult blood pressure in the 1946 British birth cohort. Lancet 362:1178–1183
40. Ghosh AK, Hardy RJ, Francis DP et al (2014) Midlife blood pressure change and left ventricular mass and remodelling in older age in the 1946 British birth cohort studydagger. Eur Heart J 35:3287–3295
41. Allen NB, Siddique J, Wilkins JT et al (2014) Blood pressure trajectories in early adulthood and subclinical atherosclerosis in middle age. JAMA 311(5):490–497
42. Ghosh AK, Hughes AD, Francis D et al (2016) Midlife blood pressure predicts future diastolic dysfunction independently of blood pressure. Heart 102:1380–1387

43. Hardy R, Cooper R, Sayer AA et al (2013) Body mass index, muscle strength and physical performance in older adults from eight cohort studies: the HALCyon programme. PLoS One 8(2):e56483
44. Singh-Manoux A, Dugravot A, Shipley M et al (2017) Obesity trajectories and risk of dementia: 28 years of follow-up in the Whitehall II Study. Alzheimers Dement 14:178–186
45. Senese LC, Almeida ND, Fath AK, Smith BT, Loucks EB (2009) Associations between childhood socioeconomic position and adulthood obesity. Epidemiol Rev 31:21–51
46. Bann D, Cooper R, Wills AK, Adams J, Kuh D (2014) Socioeconomic position across life and body composition in early old age: findings from a British birth cohort study. J Epidemiol Community Health 68(6):516–523
47. Bann D, Johnson W, Li L, Kuh D, Hardy R (2017) Socioeconomic inequalities in body mass index across adulthood: coordinated analyses of individual participant data from three British birth cohort studies initiated in 1946, 1958 and 1970. PLoS Med 14(1):e1002214
48. Johnson W, Li L, Kuh D, Hardy R (2015) How has the age-related process of overweight or obesity development changed over time? Co-ordinated analyses in five United Kingdom birth cohorts. PLoS Med 12(5):e1001828
49. Bann D, Johnson W, Kuh D, Hardy R (2018) Socioeconomic inequalities in childhood and adolescent body-mass index, weight, and height from 1953 to 2015: an analysis of four longitudinal, observational, British birth cohort studies. Lancet Public Health 3(4):e194–e203

Healthy Ageing: What Is It and How to Describe It?

2

Ritu Sadana and Jean-Pierre Michel

Key Messages

- Two approaches to define successful ageing are analysed from literature and citation patterns from 1902 to 2015: the first reflects older adults' views and the second, those of researchers and clinicians.
- In the first approach, older adults' agree that ageing is a continuous, adaptive process, whereas what is important is the ability to do what he or she values, the essence of well-being. This conceptualization aligns with WHO's definition of "Healthy Ageing" adopted by its Member States in 2016. It reflects a person-centred approach, inclusive of all older adults, not only those who are disease- or disability-free but also defined by a clinical threshold.
- A standardized approach to measure Healthy Ageing, based on a tested and comparable way to describe it (e.g. domains), measure it (e.g. measurement modes), and report on it (e.g. interpretation norms), would advance global monitoring, research, and evidence syntheses on the impact of interventions, across populations, and over time.
- New methods, technologies, and tools to measure and report on intrinsic capacities (e.g. within the body-mind) and functional ability (within one's specific environmental-social context) are urgently needed to better capture and identify the ways to optimize healthy ageing in our own environment, over the entire life course, and communicate to others what we value. This will provide a powerful and needed alternative to disease- and organ-based descriptions.

R. Sadana (✉)
Department of Ageing and Life Course, World Health Organization, Geneva, Switzerland
e-mail: sadanar@who.int

J.-P. Michel
University of Geneva, Geneva, Switzerland

French Academy of Medicine, Paris, France

J.-P. Michel (ed.), *Prevention of Chronic Diseases and Age-Related Disability*, Practical Issues in Geriatrics, https://doi.org/10.1007/978-3-319-96529-1_2

2.1 Introduction

In 2016, more than 3000 new scientific papers were devoted to "Healthy Ageing" and more than 500 were focused on "Successful Ageing." Trying to digest this prolific literature highlights the current confusion surrounding the exact meaning of, and ways to operationalize and measure these two terms. Two recent publications contribute to the current understanding of these concepts.

The first innovative contribution, by Kusumastutia and colleagues [1], offers insight on intellectual origins, as it reviews all papers on "successful ageing" from 1902 to 2015, within the Web of Science Core Collection Database. By using the CitNetExplorer software, and visualizing outcomes using timeline-based citation patterns, the analysis differentiates two distinct citation networks:

- The first, called the Havighurst cluster, contains 1146 publications and 3946 citation links, and focuses on successful ageing from the perspective of older persons themselves. Across the lifespan, the Havighurst cluster highlights the importance of the continuous, adaptive processes that adults undergo to modify their goals in the face of losses that are often gradual [1].
- The second, called the Katz cluster, has 609 publications and 1682 citation links. It views successful ageing primarily from the perspective of measurements as determined by researchers, often clinicians. According to this view, to be successful, older persons' functioning is assessed based on criteria and predetermined cut-points, usually dichotomous [1].

A recent analysis of the English Cognitive Function and Ageing Studies [2] illustrates the ongoing implications of the Havighurst–Katz distinction, that make it difficult to compare and interpret measures that reflect these distinct perspectives. The issue is which perspective should be privileged to better understand healthy ageing? Jagger et al. compare results from 1991 and 2011 of three health measures (general self-reported health; Mini Mental State Examination; and disability in activities), with health expectancies reflecting the age- and sex-specific prevalence of each health measure, in populations aged 65 and over in three English towns, Cambridge, Newcastle, and Nottingham. They report gains in life expectancy at age 65 (i.e., 4.5 years for men and 3.6 years for women) were equivalent to gains in years free of any cognitive impairment (4.2 years for men and 4.4 years for women) as well as further decreased years with mild or moderate-severe impairment. However, gains in disability-free years (2.6 years for men and only 0.5 years for women) were much smaller than gains in years with excellent or good self-reported health (3.8 years for men and 3.1 years for women), mostly due to increased mild disability [2]. Reflecting on these results from one study in a high-income country, the authors discuss these as evidence of absolute and relative compression, or at least equilibrium, of impairments, general health status, or disability, given increasing life expectancy in England.

However, that a difference exists between "disability-free" and "excellent-good health" years gained is not surprising, as the gap probably reflects the Havighurst–Katz distinction, e.g., between researchers' predetermined criteria for disability free (that requires a very high level to be "free" resulting most likely in an under-estimation of gains) and the general health status reported by the same participants (where older adults may report experiencing good health, or even good "well-being," regardless of their clinical condition, impairment, or disability) [3]. Some have labelled this phenomenon as "the disability paradox" [4]. However, as people age, it may be that "healthy ageing" reflects peoples' capacities and what they are enabled to do, and external assessments of impairment or disabilities should not be the basis to determine whether an individual is "successful" in older age.

This leads to the second publication in 2015, the WHO World Report on Ageing and Health [5], as it takes this person-centered approach, and proposes a new, more realistic and pragmatic concept of "Healthy Ageing." It also puts forth the importance of a public health response to ensure that the needs of older adults are met.

With this introduction, this chapter outlines briefly the progression of ideas, terms, definitions, and possible interpretations of what makes up "good" ageing from the latter half of the past century to the introduction of the WHO definition of "Healthy Ageing."

2.2 Brief Summary of the History of the "Ageing Concept"

The first key element in this short history is 1948 when WHO Member States adopted a new definition of health as "a state of complete physical, mental and social well-being and not merely the absence of disease or infirmity" [6]. The 1986 Ottawa Charter for Health Promotion, built on the progress made through the Declaration on Primary Health Care at Alma-Ata, and further specified that to "reach a state of complete physical, mental, and social wellbeing, an individual or group must be able to identify and to realize aspirations, to satisfy needs, and to change or cope with the environment" [7]. These fundamentals should be understood in the context of "health as the capacity to love and work" [8]; and the importance of "happiness, harmonious relations and security of all peoples" [6].

A second element is that health at both ends of the spectrum of life may be more closely related than previously thought. The life course approach [9] connects broader social, political, and environmental determinants of health, including the organization and effectiveness of health and other social systems, to health outcomes, across all critical life stages [refer to D. Kuh's chap. 1]. Along with genetic variation, the impact can explain the wide variations in the rate of ageing [10], in terms of declining capacities [9] eventually resulting in frailty, disease, disability, and death [11].

Although the promoting and maintaining of intrinsic capacity is a priority from a medical perspective, evidence indicates that what is more important to the individual, particularly older adults, is functional ability that enables a person to do what he or she values, the essence of well-being [7, 8], the third element. Specifically, WHO defines functional ability as "the health related attributes that enable people to be and to do what they have reason to value. It is determined by the intrinsic capacity of the individual (i.e., the combination of all the individual's physical and mental capacities). Intrinsic capacity at any point in time is determined by many factors, including underlying physiological and psychological changes, health-related behaviors, and the presence or absence of disease.

Objective well-being includes people's living conditions and their opportunities to realize their potential, which in principle should be equitably distributed among all people, including older adults. Moreover, three components make up subjective well-being: eudemonic well-being—self-perceptions of autonomy, competence, purpose of life, locus of control; positive and negative states—experience of joy, happiness, anxiety, sadness; and life evaluation—a reflective assessment [12]. Well-being is more than just physical health or objective living conditions, as it carries strong connotations of happiness, but also of hedonism [13].

Moreover, the benefits of maintaining "good health" well into old age include reduced dependency and healthcare costs [14]. "Good health" will allow older people to continue participating productively in society, and to put to good use the many advantages older adults can offer, such as their stability, a heightened ability to manage conflicts, and their consideration for other age groups [14].

Since mid-twentieth century, the number of attempts to name, define, conceive, and measure the process of ageing across the life span has been impressively diverse (see Table 2.1). Even when limited to literature mostly from Western and higher income country settings, different concepts and definitions reflect distinct viewpoints, norms, and values, as well as differences in the approach to measurement and interpretation [1].

Table 2.1 Key concepts in a brief history of the ageing concept (see also Martin et al. [15])

Basic healthy ageing definition	General condition of ageing of a person's mind and body, usually meaning freedom from illness, injury, or pain	
Ego integrity vs despair (1950)	Subjective evaluation of one's life as having been a fulfilling and satisfying one	Erickson [16]
Activity theory (1961)	Maintaining middle-aged activities and attitudes into later adulthood	Cumming and Henry [17]
Disengagement theory (1961)	Desire and ability of older people to disengage from active life in order to prepare themselves for death	Cumming and Henry [17]
Successful ageing (1961)	Conditions promoting a maximum of satisfaction and happiness	Havighurst [18]
Successful ageing (1963)	Having inner feelings of happiness and satisfaction with one's present and past life	Havighurst [19]
Index of activities of daily living (ADL) (1963)	Systematic approach to measuring physical performance in a population of older or chronically ill persons	Katz et al. [20]
Ageing successfully (1972)	Coping style, prior ability to adapt, and expectations of life, as well as income, health, social interactions, freedoms, and constraints; coalescence of personality which plays into the enormous complexity of successful ageing	Neugarten [21]
Successful ageing (1987; 1998)	Interplay between social engagement with life, health, and functioning for a positive ageing experience (low probability of disease and disease-related disability)	Rowe and Kahn [22, 23]

Table 2.1 (continued)

Basic healthy ageing definition	General condition of ageing of a person's mind and body, usually meaning freedom from illness, injury, or pain	
Selective optimization with compensation (1990)	(a) Selective adaptation and transformation of internal and external resources (b) optimization and compensation (c) maintenance of function, maximizing gains and minimizing losses	Baltes and Baltes [24]
Productive ageing (1990)	Any activity by an older individual that contributes to producing goods or services, or develops the capacity to produce them (whether or not the individual is paid for this activity)	Butler et al. [25]
Active ageing (2002)	Active ageing is the process of optimizing opportunities for health, participation, and security in order to enhance quality of life as people age	WHO [26]
Civic engagement (2004)	Need to involve older adults in the community, create opportunities for participation, and generate further interest in the mutual benefit of participation for community beneficiaries and participants	GSA [27]; Martinson et al. [28]
Gerotranscendence (2005)	Legacy building and existential concerns allowing old age to possess its own meaning and character	Tornstam [29]
Healthy ageing (2006)	Optimizing opportunities for good health, so that older people can take an active part in society and enjoy an independent and high quality of life	Swedish National Institute of Public Health [30]
Cultural aspects of "good ageing"(2007)	Different cultures have different understandings and interact in different ways to promote or detract from a "good old age"	Fry et al. [31]
Successful ageing and diseases (2009)	Successful ageing may coexist with diseases and functional limitations *if* compensatory psychological and/or social mechanisms are used	Young et al. [3]
Cognitive and emotional aspects of successful ageing (2010)	There is a gulf between researcher and lay definitions—the former describes freedom from disease and disability, and the latter focuses on adaptation, meaningfulness, and connection	Jeste et al. [32]
Healthy and active ageing (2011)	The process of optimizing opportunities for health to enhance quality of life as people age and grow old	European Commission [33]
Resilient ageing (2014)	The process an older person endures beyond physical, psychosocial, or cognitive adversity, through protective factors that influence the attributes of coping, hardiness, and self-concept, in the person's quest towards quality of life	Hicks and Conner [34]
Healthy ageing (2015)	Healthy ageing is more than just the absence of disease; it is the process of developing and maintaining the functional ability that enables well-being in older age	WHO [5]

Bearing in mind all these interacting factors, approaches to the concept of ageing have evolved from the disengagement theory promoted in the 1960s [17], towards a more "positive gerontology" approach, which really took off in the late 1980s [22]. Currently, the WHO's 2015 definition of "Healthy Ageing" [5] appears to be most realistic, and considers continuous, trajectories of health across the life course, rather than a focus on chronologic age or a threshold for good ageing [10]. It is also more realistic as it is inclusive of all older adults, in contrast to "successful ageing" or "anti-ageing" discourses that focus on elimination of disease or ageing processes. It is also more visionary, as it recognizes all older adults, irrespective of their level of intrinsic capacities, can be supported to have a good level of functional ability.

2.3 The New WHO Definition of Healthy Ageing

In the preface to the first World Report on Ageing and Health, WHO's Director-General clearly states that "healthy ageing is more than just the absence of disease" [5]. The new definition of Healthy Ageing proposed in the Report and in the first WHO Global Strategy and Action Plan on Ageing and Health [35], unanimously endorsed by all WHO Member States during the World Health Assembly in May 2016, is "the process of developing and maintaining functional ability that enables well-being in older age." While the definition reflects what older adults value, the approach to classify, measure, and improve it is linked to the WHO International Classification of Functioning (ICF) [36, 37], as it recognizes the ongoing interaction between an individual and their environment:

- Each individual has their own "intrinsic capacity," resulting from the complex interaction between their genetic inheritance, personal and health characteristics, including age-related physiological changes, risk factor accumulation, and impact of acute or chronic clinical conditions. Indeed, personal intellectual potential, as well as psychological adaptation and resilience across the life course, modify capacity. In summary, "intrinsic capacity" is the composite of all individual, physical, and mental capacities.
- Each individual lives in a specific environment, that can change over time, and is highly dependent on political, economic, and social norms, values, and resources, including the extent that societies promote equal opportunities, prevent inequities, and combat ageism, and indeed, ensure access to affordable health and social systems. The close interactions between intrinsic capacity and environmental characteristics (including surroundings itself and support) combine to determine "functional ability."

Moreover, differences in older adults' health and illness experiences to a large extent reflect accumulated inequalities across peoples' lives. When unfair, these are called health inequities, and are considered "avoidable, unfair and unjust" and exist within and across countries, from high to low resources settings [refer to R. Sadana's chap. 18].

The implication is that the life span trajectories of intrinsic capacity (IC) and functional ability (FA), which can be similar during the first part of life in a hospitable environment, start to diverge in midlife with the impact of accumulated determinants of health, and the onset of declines in intrinsic capacities. The increasing decline in intrinsic capacity with time is more or less compensated by support and surroundings reflecting a person's specific environment. Yet an imbalance between the needs of an individual and an environment that does not address, fulfill, or compensate these needs, partly contributing to care dependence and resulting in decreased functional ability and overall well-being.

The World Report on Ageing and Health, and the accompanying Global Strategy, outline evidence and actions towards optimizing intrinsic capacity and functional ability particularly during the second part of life, allowing older adults to do things that are important for them [5].

This innovative life course approach is extremely interesting because it brings together in a single public health concept both previously described perspectives on ageing, namely the viewpoint of older adults and the clinician-researchers' approaches to address important declines or care dependency, through its public health framework [1] (see Fig. 2.1).

Figure 2.1 illustrates conceptually that when considering the population as a whole, IC and FA can vary across the second half of the life course. Trajectories reflect a continuous phenomenon and can be divided into three common periods: a

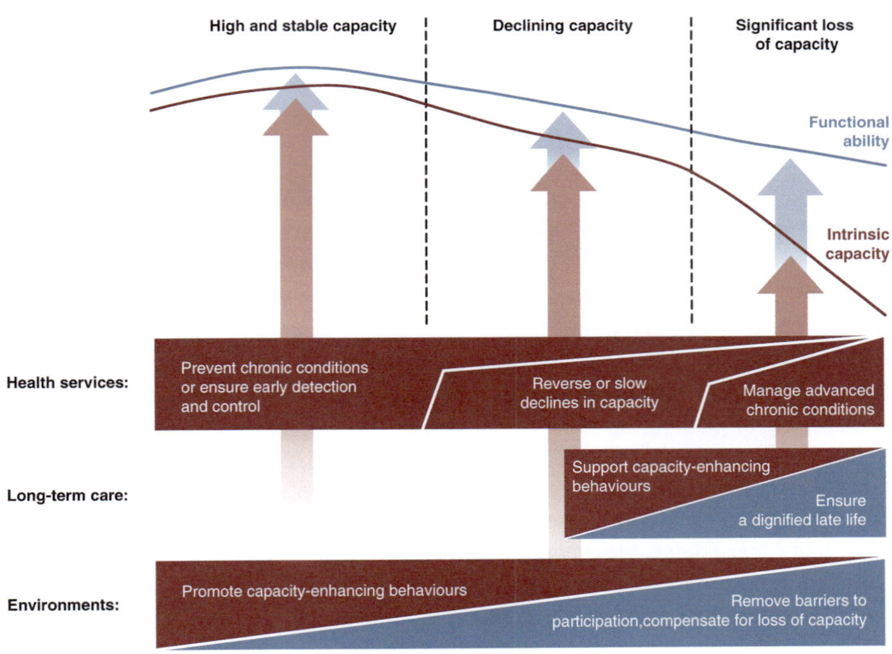

Fig. 2.1 Public health framework for Healthy Ageing: opportunities for action across the life course, reproduced from WHO 2015

period of relatively high and stable capacity, a period of declining capacity, and a period of significant loss of capacity. These periods are not defined by chronological age and trajectories are not necessarily monotonic (i.e., continually decreasing). Distinguishing between IC and FA is necessary in order to understand if levels, distributions, and trajectories of functioning are due to changes in the individual or the environments they inhabit. It is also necessary in order to document what can be done to improve IC and FA for individuals, groups or populations, involving different policies, sectors, and interventions.

The WHO Global Strategy and Action Plan and other recent publications outlines several strategic areas to transform the health services delivery systems from disease-centered practice to a more integrated conception of care from birth to very old age, coordinated across providers, favoring the highest intrinsic capacity and indeed functional ability, by placing functioning evaluation and maintenance as the first priority [38].

Two major questions emerge from this concept: the first is, what public health approach can be used to achieve the appropriate system of health and social care (see the WHO Report) [5]. This includes how best to design and evaluate interventions to facilitate healthy ageing and decrease/delay if not reverse the declines in capacity or ability, which are the two sides of the same coin. Numerous intervention studies have been performed, but have all focused on specific aspects of ageing [39] and not on the whole integrated process, which would be more in line with the new concept of healthy ageing [40–45]. The second is how can we measure the life trajectories of intrinsic capacity and functional ability, discussed next.

2.4 Measurements of Ageing: Towards a Standardized Approach

This issue remains unresolved. The approach to measurement should reflect the concept, agreement on how to operationalize it, and then identify specific measures, tests, questions, assessments, etc., that yields valid and reliable results, fit for purpose, for each life stage, and across the life course. Given the Havighurst–Katz distinction, it is not surprising that current efforts to assess health outcomes for older adults draw on four categories: items reflecting the WHO definition of health and well-being; symptom oriented or considered indicative of illness or morbidity; on fulfilling or performing functions, activities, or roles (such as activities of daily living—ADLs or IADLs); and those concerned with adaptation or coping with conditions or limitations [46]. Many standardized instruments exit, whether for the general population, specific diseases or condition, or specific population sub-groups, including older adults. Most combine information on biomarkers, measured tests, capacity to perform tasks, and subjective evaluation. Data collected through these instruments are often presented as multiple dimensional profiles. An overview of ten recent approaches to assess older adults (see Table 2.2) illustrates each uses different domains, with different elements listed within each domain. Not shown is that each includes different items, recall periods, response scales, and proposed

Table 2.2 Compilation of the different domains used to describe ageing in ten recently published studies

	Phelan and Larson [47]	Young et al. [3]	Sabia et al. [48]	Tyrovolas et al. [49]	Bousquet et al. [50]	Cosco et al. [51]	Lara et al. [52]	Assmann et al. [53]	Tampubolon [54]	Jaspers et al. [55]
Education				X						
Diet				X						
Physiological/Physical Health					X					
Nl function/markers		X	X				X			X
CVx			X	X			X			
Lung/respiratory			X						X	
Metabolic				X			X		X	
Endocrine							X		X	
Musculo-Skeletal		X	X							
Inflammation							X	X	X	X
No Chronic Disease (CVx, COPD, Cancer, diabetes)					X				X	X
No pain								X	X	
Mental Health										
Intact cognition			XX		X	X	X	X	X	X
Good mood/emotion		X	X	X	X			X	X	X
Preserved autonomy			X							X
Daily Functioning					X					
No ADL inability	X				X	X		X	X	
Functional independence	X						X			
Walking speed			X		X		X			
FEV1			X				X			

(continued)

Table 2.2 (continued)

	Phelan and Larson [47]	Young et al. [3]	Sabia et al. [48]	Tyrovolas et al. [49]	Bousquet et al. [50]	Cosco et al. [51]	Lara et al. [52]	Assmann et al. [53]	Tampubolon [54]	Jaspers et al. [55]
Personal perception										
Feeling								X	X	
Resource						X				
Engagement	X	X			X		X			
Goals	X									
Satisfaction	X									
Quality of Life	X				X					X
Social life								X		
Activities participation	X			X	X				X	
Support										X
Relations					X					
Spirituality		X							X	
Wealth				X						
Environment										
Healthy					X					
Controlled										

cut-offs to categorize individuals. None listed have produced sufficient assessments that would document trajectories across the entire life course, or link clinical assessments with community- or population-based monitoring.

However, the many high quality longitudinal studies such as those within the Health and Retirement Studies family [56] in a growing number of countries offer an opportunity to help the scientific community to better apprehend the complex interactions and challenges of human ageing, whether at the individual or population level [57–59]. Nonetheless, the different measurement approaches used to describe and assess ageing do not enable a clear assessment of progress in a comparable way over time or across countries [1]—this is very disappointing.

This is so as currently there is no reference criterion for assessing healthy ageing [52]. Consequently, it is difficult to conduct and compare research and descriptions of ageing across studies [60]. In order to agree on ways to describe, measure, analyze, and monitor IC and FA, each concept requires further clarification, including a description of what are its components (see Box 2.1), pathways to optimize each across the life course, measurement approaches, and useful metrics to monitor and communicate progress.

Box 2.1

Previous efforts within WHO to measure health through multi-dimensional profiles have been guided by the following key criteria:

- valid in terms of intuitive, clinical, and epidemiological concepts of health
- linked to the conceptual framework of the ICF International Classification of Functioning, Disability and Health
- amenable to self-report, observation, or direct measurement
- comprehensive enough to capture the most important aspects of health states that people value
- cross-population comparable

Innovative approaches and technologies are urgently needed to conceive new tools to enable us to better capture what happens to our body in our own environment, where we live, over the whole life course, and communicate to others what we value. This information will allow individuals to play an active role in preserving their capacities and abilities, become actors of health promotion and care management, and make decisions informed by what they value.

Acknowledgments RS is a staff member of the World Health Organization and along with JPM is alone responsible for the views expressed in this publication; these do not necessarily represent the decisions, policy, or views of the World Health Organization. This chapter is based on an article published in JAMDA 2017; 18: 460–4.

Declaration of Interest: JPM and RS are co-authors, with others, of the WHO Report on Ageing and Health 2015.

References

1. Kusumastutia S, Derksb MGL, Tellier S, Di Nucci E, Lund R, Mortensen EL, Westendorp RGJ (2016) Successful ageing: a study of the literature using citation network analysis. Maturitas 93:4–12
2. Jagger C, Matthews FE, Wohland P et al (2016) A comparison of health expectancies over two decades in England: results of the Cognitive Function and Ageing Study I and II. Lancet 387:779–786
3. Young Y, Frick KD, Phelan EA (2009) Can successful aging and chronic illness coexist in the same individual? A multidimensional concept of successful aging. J Am Med Dir Assoc 10:87–92
4. Albrecht GL, Devlieger PJ (1999) The disability paradox: high quality of life against all odds. Soc Sci Med 48:977–988
5. World Health Organization (2015) World report on ageing and health. WHO, Geneva
6. World Health Organization (1948) Constitution of the World Health Organization. WHO, Geneva
7. World Health Organization (1986) Ottawa Charter for Health Promotion. WHO, Geneva
8. Smith R (2008) The end of disease and the beginning of health. TheBMJopinion. https://blogs.bmj.com/bmj/2008/07/08/richard-smith-the-end-of-disease-and-the-beginning-of-health/. Accessed 17 Apr 2017
9. Hanson MA, Cooper C, Aihie Sayer A, Eendebak RJ, Clough GF, Beard JR (2016) Developmental aspects of a life course approach to healthy ageing. J Physiol 594:2147–2160
10. Sadana R, Blas E, Budhwani S, Koller T, Paraje G (2016) Healthy ageing: raising awareness of inequalities, determinants, and what could be done to improve health equity. Gerontologist 56(Suppl 2):S178–S193
11. Mount S, Lara J, Schols AM, Mathers JC (2016) Towards a multidimensional healthy ageing phenotype. Curr Opin Clin Nutr Metab Care 19:418–426
12. World Health Organization Regional Office for Europe (2012) Charting the way to well-being. World Health Organization Regional Office for Europe, Copenhagen
13. Brussow H (2013) What is health? Microb Biotechnol 6:341–348
14. Rowe JW, Kahn RL (2015) Successful aging 2.0: conceptual expansions for the 21st century. J Gerontol B Psychol Sci Soc Sci 70:593–596
15. Martin P, Kelly N, Kahana B et al (2015) Defining successful aging: a tangible or elusive concept? Gerontologist 55:14–25
16. Erikson EH (1950) Childhood and society. Norton, New York
17. Cumming E, Henry WE (1961) Growing old: the process of disengagement. Basic Books, New York
18. Havighurst RJ (1961) Successful aging. The Gerontologist 1:8–13
19. Havighurst RJ (1963) Successful aging. In: Williams rH, Tibbitts C, Donahue W (eds) Processes of aging. Atherton Press, New York, pp 299–320
20. Katz S, Ford AB, Moskowitz RW, Jackson BA, Jaffe MW (1963) Studies of illness in the aged. The index of Adl: a standardized measure of biological and psychosocial function. JAMA 185:914–919
21. Neugarten BL (1972) Personality and the aging process. Gerontologist 12:9–15
22. Rowe JW, Kahn RL (1987) Human aging: usual and successful. Science 237:143–149
23. Rowe JW, Kahn RL (1998) Successful aging. Aging (Milano) 10:142–144
24. Baltes PB, Baltes MM (1990) Successful aging: perspectives from the behavioral sciences. Cambridge University Press, Cambridge
25. Butler R, Oberlink M, Schecter M (1990) The promise of productive aging. Springer, New York
26. World Health Organization (WHO) (2002) Active ageing: a policy framework. World Health Organization, Geneva
27. Press release: civic engagemnent of in an older America. 2004. http://www.civicengagement.org/agingsociety/Pages%20from%20Geron-NLSept05.pdf. Accessed 4 Feb 2017

28. Martinson M, Minkler M (2006) Civic engagement and older adults: a critical perspective. Gerontologist 46:318–324
29. Tornstam L (2005) Gerotranscendence: a developmental theory of positive aging. Springer Publishing Company, New York
30. Swedish National Institute of Public Health. Healthy ageing: a challenge for Europe 2006
31. Fry CL, Dickerson-Putman J, Draper P, Ikels C, Keith J, Glascock P, Harpending HC (2007) Culture and the meaning of a good old age. In: Sokolovsky J (ed) The cultural context of aging: worldwide perspectives. Bergin & Garvey, Westport, CT, p 104
32. Jeste DV, Depp CA, Vahia IV (2010) Successful cognitive and emotional aging. World Psychiatry 9:78–84
33. European Commission (2011) How to promote active ageing in Europe: EU support to local and regional actors. European Commission, European Union-Committee of the Regions & Ageplatform Europe, Brussels
34. Hicks MM, Conner NE (2014) Resilient ageing: a concept analysis. J Adv Nurs 70:744–755
35. World Health Organization (2016) WHO global strategy and action plan on ageing and health (2016–2020). WHO, Geneva
36. World Health Organisation (2001) The international classification of functioning, disability and health (ICF). WHO, Geneva
37. Üstün TB, Kostanjsek N, Chatterji S, Rehm J (2010) Measuring health and disability manual for WHO disability assessment schedule WHODAS 2.0. WHO, Geneva
38. Kuruvilla S, Sadana R, Villar Montesinos E et al (2018) A life-course approach to health: synergy with sustainable development goals. Bull World Health Organ 96:42–50
39. Michel J-P, Dreux C, Vacheron A (2016) Healthy ageing: evidence that improvement is possible at every age. Eur Geriatr Med 7(4):298–305
40. Chen L-K (2016) Towards the life course approach of healthy aging. Eur Geriatr Med 7:289–290
41. Strandberg T (2016) Healthy ageing: evidence that improvement is possible at every age. Eur Geriatr Med 7:293–294
42. Barbagallo M, Dominguez LJ (2016) Healthy ageing: from a myth to a reality. Eur Geriatr Med 7:298
43. Friedman SM (2016) Response to "Healthy ageing: evidence that improvement is possible at every age". Eur Geriatr Med 7:295
44. Arai H (2016) Response to "Healthy ageing: evidence that improvement is possible at every age". Eur Geriatr Med 7:296
45. Sadana R (2016) Commentary on "Healthy ageing: evidence that improvement is possible at every age". Eur Geriatr Med 7:291–292
46. Sadana R (2002) Development of standardized health state descriptions. World Health Organization, Geneva
47. Phelan EA, Larson EB (2002) "Successful aging"—where next? J Am Geriatr Soc 50:1306–1308
48. Sabia S, Singh-Manoux A, Hagger-Johnson G, Cambois E, Brunner EJ, Kivimaki M (2012) Influence of individual and combined healthy behaviours on successful aging. CMAJ 184:1985–1992
49. Tyrovolas S, Haro JM, Mariolis A et al (2014) Successful aging, dietary habits and health status of elderly individuals: a k-dimensional approach within the multi-national MEDIS study. Exp Gerontol 60:57–63
50. Bousquet J, Kuh D, Bewick M et al (2015) Operational definition of active and healthy ageing (AHA): a conceptual framework. J Nutr Health Aging 19:955–960
51. Cosco TD, Stephan BC, Brayne C (2015) Validation of an a priori, index model of successful aging in a population-based cohort study: the successful aging index. Int Psychogeriatr 27:1971–1977
52. Lara J, Cooper R, Nissan J et al (2015) A proposed panel of biomarkers of healthy ageing. BMC Med 13:222

53. Assmann KE, Andreeva VA, Camilleri GM et al (2016) Dietary scores at midlife and healthy ageing in a French prospective cohort. Br J Nutr 116:666–676
54. Tampubolon G (2016) Trajectories of the healthy ageing phenotype among middle-aged and older Britons, 2004-2013. Maturitas 88:9–15
55. Jaspers L, Schoufour JD, Erler NS et al (2017) Development of a healthy aging score in the population-based Rotterdam study: evaluating age and sex differences. J Am Med Dir Assoc 18:276.e1
56. Gateway to global aging data, produced by the Program on Global Aging, Health & Policy, University of Southern California with funding from the National Institute on Aging (R01 AG030153) A platform for population survey data on aging and health. https://g2aging.org/. Accessed 29 Dec 2017
57. Bann D, Johnson W, Li L, Kuh D, Hardy R (2017) Socioeconomic inequalities in body mass index across adulthood: coordinated analyses of individual participant data from three British birth cohort studies initiated in 1946, 1958 and 1970. PLoS Med 14:e1002214
58. Hagger-Johnson G, Carr E, Murray E, Stansfeld S, Shelton N, Stafford M, Head J (2017) Association between midlife health behaviours and transitions out of employment from midlife to early old age: Whitehall II cohort study. BMC Public Health 17:82
59. Stafford M, Cooper R, Cadar D et al (2017) Physical and cognitive capability in mid-adulthood as determinants of retirement and extended working life in a British cohort study. Scand J Work Environ Health 43:15–23
60. Fabbri E, Zoli M, Gonzalez-Freire M, Salive ME, Studenski SA, Ferrucci L (2015) Aging and multimorbidity: new tasks, priorities, and frontiers for integrated gerontological and clinical research. J Am Med Dir Assoc 16:640–647

Midlife Prevention for a Healthy Mouth and Dentition

3

Frauke Müller

Key Messages

- A healthy mouth and dentition are integral part of the general health and well-being.
- The major oral diseases that occur in adult persons are chronic, progressive, and cumulative over the course of life.
- Causes for oral disease are closely related to lifestyles, which include a diet rich in sugar, and the use of tobacco and consumption of alcohol.
- Oral health, tooth loss, and the ageing process are often overshadowed by the social determinants of health, be it the level of education or socio-economic status.
- Despite progress in prevention and treatment techniques, oral disease remains a major public health burden.

3.1 Introduction

A healthy mouth and dentition are integral part of the general health and well-being [1]. The major oral diseases that occur in adult persons are chronic, progressive, and cumulative over the course of life. Causes for oral disease are closely related to lifestyles, which include a diet rich in sugar, and the use of tobacco and consumption of alcohol [2]. Oral infections, especially periodontal diseases, may negatively

F. Müller
Department of Internal Medicine, Rehabilitation and Geriatrics, Service of Geriatrics, University Hospitals of Geneva, Geneva, Switzerland

Division of Gerodontology and Removable Prosthodontics, University Clinics of Dental Medicine, University of Geneva, Geneva, Switzerland
e-mail: Frauke.mueller@unige.ch

J.-P. Michel (ed.), *Prevention of Chronic Diseases and Age-Related Disability*, Practical Issues in Geriatrics, https://doi.org/10.1007/978-3-319-96529-1_3

impact the general health, and associations with cardio-vascular disease, diabetes, premature birth, and bacterial pneumonia have been reported [3]. The recent trend of retaining a full or partial natural dentition until late in life has been welcomed as a sign of improving dental health, but a high prevalence of caries, periodontal disease occur along with tooth retention and continue to be a considerable public health challenge [4]. Other diseases of the oral tissues comprise a large range of mucosal conditions, as well as oropharyngeal squamous cell carcinomas, of which the prevalence steadily increases beyond the age of 60 years [5]. Finally, oral health, tooth loss, and the ageing process are often overshadowed by the social determinants of health, be it the level of education or socio-economic status. Major oral diseases affect primarily persons who are poor, disadvantaged, and/or socially deprived. Despite progress in prevention and treatment techniques, oral disease remains a major public health burden. It is important to integrate oral health into global health agenda using the common risk factor approach [6]. Although health promotion and disease prevention should be addressed in a global a multidisciplinary approach, this chapter will focus on the individual midlife measures, that any person could adopt to prevent oral disease and maintain oral health until late in life.

3.2 What Effect Has Physiological Ageing on the Orofacial System?

Most structures and functions of the orofacial system are subject to ageing, and this process is general, irreversible, and progressive. All orofacial muscles will atrophy and become thinner, especially when not trained regularly, due to tooth loss or poor dental restorations. For example, the masseter muscle, which is one of the main jaw-closing muscles, will lose 40% of its muscle bulk over the lifetime [7]. The ageing processes in the muscles include also the motor units, which become larger as individual motor fibres disappear and some muscle fibres are adopted by neighbouring motor units, hence the mandibular movements and the corresponding closing trajectories become more erratic. The salivary glands will lose some of their acinary cells, which are replaced by connective tissues. Consequently, the maximum amount of saliva produced is diminished with age. Saliva has several very important roles: it moistens the oral cavity, helps initial digesting of food and wrapping it to a coherent bolus which is safe for swallowing. It further buffers the pH in the mouth and dilutes tastes. Another function of the saliva is the protection of the mucosa and teeth. Saturated with calcium phosphate, saliva has the capacity to remineralize initial carious lesions and render a filling therapy unnecessary. Saliva from the parotid gland can be stimulated by unilateral chewing, but the maximum amount produced is declining with age. Nevertheless, the amount of saliva that is necessary to keep the mouth healthy should still be available in healthy elder adults. The high percentage of elder persons who perceive the sensation of a dry mouth is more related to underlying pathology or the side effects of their treatment [8]. With age, the oral mucosa becomes thinner and more vulnerable to mechanical injury. Major signs of ageing concern also the nervous system, which presents in elders with a reduced neuroplasticity. This implies that any changes in the oral cavity, like new dental prostheses, are less quickly adapted and the CNS struggles to create new motor patterns which corresponds to the novel restoration [9]. Ageing also touches the motor-coordination, including the complex motor patterns that are required for the swallowing reflex. About one third of elders present with swallowing disorders. Other age-related changes of the orofacial system concern the bony tissues, which present with a thinner cortical bone and a flattened articular tuberculum in the temporo-mandibular joint. The latter is present in elders with more degenerative diseases and more freedom in movement, along with the loosening of the ligaments. Last but not least, physiological ageing concerns also the natural dentition. Aged teeth appear darker, with a rather mat surface and show irregularities, signs of wear and attrition [10]. The pulpal chamber becomes smaller as secondary dentine is produced, which lowers the sensory threshold to thermal, nociceptive, and mechanical stimuli. From a functional point of view, the teeth become more brittle and less resistant to traumas such as preparation for crowns or the load from a partial denture, when they serve as abutment teeth. Teeth are meant to last for a lifetime, and although the prevalence of tooth loss increases with age, this is rather due to an accumulation of sequelae from periodontal disease and caries over the life course.

3.3 Oral Health Challenges in Old Age

The most prevalent oral conditions in old age remain coronal and root caries as well as periodontal disease, and all of them foster tooth loss when left to progress without treatment [2, 11]. Tooth loss impairs most oral functions, especially the chewing efficiency, which leads, often unconsciously, to the adoption of an unhealthy diet, as food choices are limited to what is easy to chew with few natural teeth and/or dental prostheses [12]. The daily calorie intake is often assured by a diet rich in refined carbohydrates and sugar, which provides the required calories, but lacks important nutrients like protein, vitamins, and calcium [11, 13]. Malnutrition renders elderly persons more frail and prone to disease. In old age, an elevated BMI is in general associated with a low morbidity and mortality [14]. However, the association between weight and dental state is not a direct one, as diet is strongly dominated by habits and taste preference. Improving the chewing efficiency could only indirectly improve the nutritional state, by allowing for the intake of a larger range of food stuffs, by providing the ability to eat unmixed, appetizingly looking dishes and by fostering meals in company of others, which leads to a 20% increased intake of calories [15]. Improving the dietary intake after a dental restoration with an improved chewing efficiency is not automatic, nutritional counselling is necessary to benefit from the dental intervention [16].

Another oral health challenge in old age arises from chronic diseases or their treatment. According to the WHO report on ageing, the seven most common chronic conditions in old age are cardio-vascular disease, cancer, respiratory diseases, diabetes, cirrhosis of the liver, osteoarthritis, and neurocognitive disorder [17]. Whereas diabetes has a direct negative effect on periodontal health, other diseases have a rather indirect effect on oral health, be it through the intake of medications, radiation, or chemotherapy. An undesired effect of these medications may be the sensation of a dry mouth, leading to problems in chewing, swallowing, speaking, denture wearing, and sensitivity of the mucosa [8]. When natural teeth are still present, a high risk of caries and an increase of abrasion are associated with a lack of saliva. An impaired oral health may also arise from the difficulties to perform the required oral hygiene measures, as for example in osteoarthritis and stroke, or the cognitive decline and dyspraxia as in neurocognitive disorders such as dementia.

3.4 Oral Hygiene in Old Age Is Often Poor

Oral hygiene is often poor in old age, and several reasons may account for this phenomenon [18]. Physiological ageing, which deteriorates vision, tactile sensitivity, smell and dexterity, becomes impaired in elders, even when ageing in good health. These physiological impairments render the performance of oral hygiene measures difficult. Adequate tools, like toothbrushes with thickened handles, a magnifying mirror and glasses or special tools for denture cleansing may help improving oral and denture hygiene, but their prevalence is low, and their use is not widespread custom. The natural full dentition of a young adult has a morphology that fosters self-cleaning of the oral cavity during chewing. The interdental spaces are filled with gingival papillae, and the teeth are shaped in a way, that food glides into the oral vestibule, thus protecting the delicate gingival margin from food impaction. The palate presents with rugae, which helps pushing the food into the tongue in a way that enables the taste sensation from the gustatory papillae, which are located in the depths of the tongue surface. Palatal rugae also help cleaning the tongue by providing a rough surface against which the tongue can rub against for cleaning. With time, sequalae of dental disease accumulate, and often the interdental papillae present recessions leaving the morphology of the dentition with niches where food and dental plaque can adhere without being disturbed by the cheek or the tongue (Figs. 3.1 and 3.2). Another age-related factor is the use of lower muscles forces

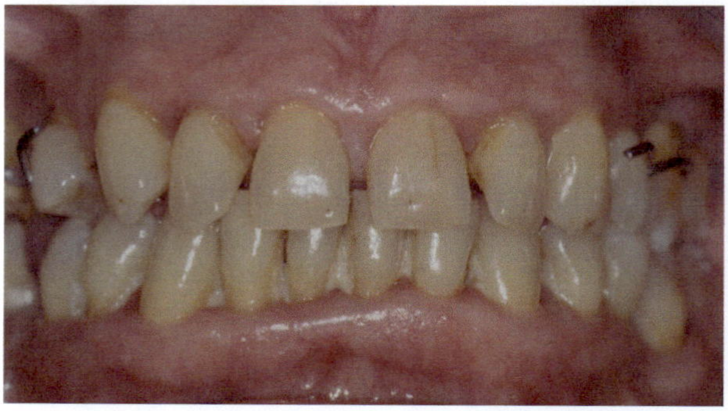

Fig. 3.1 Spaces between the incisor teeth indicate a loss of anchorage of the teeth in their bony sockets due to a chronic periodontal disease. Between the lower incisors, massive dental plaque has accumulated

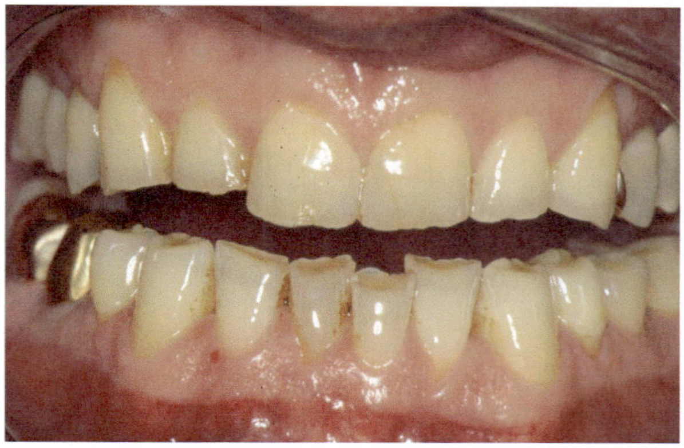

Fig. 3.2 Signs of ageing will always occur in a dentition, but teeth are meant to last for a lifetime

during mastication, such as the tongue, cheek, and lip forces, which lead to a lower self-cleaning of the oral cavity during mastication. Oral hygiene may also become painful when medication-induced hyposalivation renders the oral mucosa sensitive and painful, as the protective and repairing effects of saliva are missing. This pain exacerbates under radio- or chemotherapy as used in treating cancer.

Another reason for poor oral hygiene may be a shift in priorities, when chronic diseases and functional impairment dominate daily life. Last but not least the withdrawal from social life implies a diminished pressure for a well-tended appearance, including a "fresh breath". When living an institutionalized context, with little social interaction, and often little "secret" about the presence of a removable prostheses, the threshold to not wearing a (potentially uncomfortable) prosthesis or to not brushing the teeth is low.

3.5 What Preventive Measures Can Be Implemented in Midlife to Facilitate a Healthy Mouth and Dentition Until Late in Life?

In oral health, more than in any other discipline of medicine, prevention is the key to healthy oral ageing. Many oral diseases have known risk factors, or at least strong associations are reported. Although a public health approach to prevent oral disease has been recommended earlier in this chapter, there are a number of individual preventive measures, which any midlife adult person could adopt.

3.5.1 Alcohol and Smoking

Smoking and alcohol abuse are well-documented risk factors for oral cancer, and in addition, the oral squamous cell carcinomas have an increasing prevalence beyond the age of 60 years. Smoking is equally a recognized risk factor for periodontal diseases, be it the acute necrotic ulcerative gingivitis, also called "Gauloise-type", or the rather chronic forms of adult periodontal disease [19]. Smoking cessation is also recommended when implant placement is planned, as implant survival shows lower rates in patients who smoke.

3.5.2 Diet

Diet also plays a role in prevention of oral diseases. A diet low in calcium and vitamins may negatively impact the periodontal health and finally lead to tooth loss. The most efficient prevention for coronal and root caries is a diet low in sugar and acids. It is the combination of sugar, bacteria, and certain host factors that trigger the demineralization of the dental enamel. If left untreated, the acids are creating carious cavities, which progress rapidly towards the dentin, once the densely mineralized enamel is trespassed. When finally reaching the pulp, vivid pain signals the infection, which can penetrate through the apical foramen and spread to the alveolar bone.

3.5.3 Oral Hygiene

The most well-documented prevention in dentistry is the removal of oral biofilm, which forms with time on hard objects, such as teeth and dentures in the oral cavity. Oral biofilm consists of micro-organisms and their products embedded in an intercellular matrix. Regular disruption of biofilm is imperative for prevention and management of oral diseases, although genetic factors, as well as the individual composition of the oral microbial flora may equally play a role. Professional oral hygiene cleans the oral cavity beyond what is possible with personal oral hygiene measures. Tartar is mostly located opposing the glandular output, that is vestibular of the upper first molar and lingual of the lower incisors. It is supra-gingivally located calcified dental plaque, which cannot be removed by simple tooth brushing. Similarly calcified deposits are located on the root surface within gingival pockets, which can also not be removed by means of a tooth brush. Scaling and root planning with special ultrasound tools or sharpened instruments are used to remove these deposits from the periodontal pockets and the infected cementum from the root surface, which subsequently allows the inflamed gingival tissues to heal.

3.5.4 Application of Fluoride

The development of carious lesions is based on a process of demineralization of the dental enamel. Application of fluorides strengthens the enamel against the attacks of acids produced from bacteria out of sugary substrates. Various forms of fluoride application exist, with water fluoridation being the first population-based approach that proved successful in the reduction of caries. Contemporary standard toothpastes contain 1450 ppm of fluoride, but stronger concentrations exist with 5000 ppm, a formula that is available only on prescription. The latter toothpastes are used for a 3–6 months period to prevent root caries and even inactivate existing active root caries lesions. Other forms of fluoride application comprise varnishes, gels, and mouth rinses, mostly applied during professional oral hygiene sessions.

3.5.5 Prevention of Technical Failure

When dental restorations, be they fillings, crowns and fixed bridges or removable partial or complete dental prostheses are present, regular technical check-ups are part of the recommended preventive scheme. These check-ups aim to examine whether the dental prostheses efficiently fulfil the restoration of oral functions without any harm to the orofacial system, but also investigate the integrity of the material, abrasion, surface roughness, porosity, corrosion, fissures, and defects. Fillings with over-contoured borders foster adhesion of biofilm and hence the development of carious lesions at the tooth-filling interface. These restorations need to be corrected or replaced, in order to improve the self-cleaning morphology of the dentition. Prevention in midlife adulthood comprises a comprehensive assessment of the viability of the residual dentition and its dental restorations, with the perspective of a future functional decline, which may render the cleaning of a less than perfect restoration impossible, even when in midlife adulthood, the challenge can still be effectively managed. Given the possibility of biological and pathological complications in old age, it seems reasonable to prevent as much as possible technical failure of dental restorations by using state-of-the-art techniques and well-documented biomaterials.

3.5.6 Uptake of Dental Services

Periodic recall at the dentist and professional oral hygiene, performed by a dental hygienist or another trained dental professional, contributes to preventing oral disease. These recall visits serve screening of the oral mucosa for cancer or other diseases, but aim also for the detection of initial caries and the examination of the periodontal tissues for clinical signs of inflammation, notably swelling, bleeding, redness, and increased periodontal pocket depth. If dental restorations are already present, these need regular maintenance to remain in function and not present niches or surface defects. Check-ups further comprise the assessment of the firm seating of a prosthesis and the occlusion between the upper and lower teeth to assure oral comfort and prevent dysfunction of the temporo-mandibular articulations. The recall intervals are determined according to the individual risk of the patient, be it an elevated risk for caries or periodontal disease, chronic diseases, medication intake, lack of saliva, radio- and chemotherapy, and/or the presence of dental restorations. Preventive measures also largely depend on the functional independence and cognitive performance of the patient. In midlife adulthood, prevention consists of instruction and motivation for oral hygiene. In slightly dependent elders, this extends to supervision and control, and when further functional decline occurs prevention comprises the assistance for oral hygiene measures. Once a person's autonomy is lost, the responsibility for oral hygiene measures lies with the caring staff, who performs the necessary gestures on behalf of the patient.

3.5.7 Oral Health Care Plan

In midlife, well before the onset of frailty, but at latest at a pre-frail stage, patient and dentist should together establish an oral health care plan, the aim of which is to establish a home-care plan to prevent and control oral disease, control pain and infection, eliminate dysfunction, and assure a good oral health-related quality of life [20]. This plan includes the explanation of the risk factors for oral disease and incentive risk modification behaviour, like cessation of smoking, moderate alcohol intake, a healthy diet, and regular uptake of dental services. The intake of Vitamin D and Calcium, at doses that aim to prevent osteoporosis, is effective in reducing tooth loss [21]. The oral health care plan explains also the implications of increasing dependency on oral healthcare and specific treatment outcomes, especially involving complicated oral prostheses. The associated risk assessment includes identifying conditions threatening oral health and evinces particular risk for caries and periodontal disease, for example, a low salivary flow rate, in order to agree on the appropriate periodic recalls. It should further determine customized set of oral hygiene tools, adapted to the dentition, but also to functional impairments like impaired vision, low hand force, and dexterity [22].

3.5.8 Prevention at the Onset of Frailty and Multimorbidity

Along with the onset of frailty and functional decline, a wider inter-professional health care team will deliver various care plans, and the oral health care plan should be integrated part of this Scheme [23]. For the prevention of periodontal disease, antibacterial toothpastes should be recommended along with professional oral hygiene sessions. Chlorhexidine products may temporarily be used to control infection [24]. At the frailty stage, prevention extends to avoiding aspiration pneumonia, a frequent disease in institutionalized patients, especially those with swallowing disorders. One in ten deaths from pneumonia is prevented by weekly professional oral hygiene, when performed by a dental health professional [25, 26]. Denture wearing during the night equally doubles the incidence of pneumonia, hence frail elders should refrain from wearing their removable appliances during the night, as their bacterial load present a health hazard in terms of pneumonia [27]. It is recommended to store those removable prostheses dry when sleeping, so that bacteria are dead before the denture is cleaned and re-inserted the next morning [28]. At this stage, it is also advisable to assess the adverse effects from polypharmacy, such as hyposalivation and sugar in medications, mostly syrups [29, 30]. Relief from dry mouth is provided from water spray in an atomizer bottle, unilateral chewing activities (gum or chewy tubes), or finally salivary substitutes which come in forms of sprays, gels, or mouthrinses [31]. Besides establishing an oral health care plan, the oral health care professional's role is to inform and educate the patient on preventive measures and monitor their effectiveness.

3.6 Summary and Conclusion

Most risk factors for oral disease and tooth loss can be avoided by managing the related risk factors, notably a healthy diet, daily meticulous oral hygiene, moderate alcohol intake, and smoking cessation. Dental restorations should be state of the art and made from biocompatible, well-documented materials to avoid iatrogenic biological and technical complications. Genetics, socio-economic context and further, yet undocumented risks, may equally play a role in the development of oral disease and tooth loss.

References

1. WHO (2003) The world health report 2003—shaping the future. World Health Organization, Geneva
2. Petersen PE, Bourgeois D, Ogawa H et al (2005) The global burden of oral disease and risks to oral health. WHO, Geneva
3. Li X, Kolltveit KM, Tronstad L, Olsen I (2016) Systemic diseases caused by oral infection. Clin Microbiol Rev 13:547–558
4. Hayes M, Da Mata C, Cole M et al (2016) Risk indicators associated with root caries in independently living older adults. J Dent 51:8–14. https://doi.org/10.1016/j.jdent.2016.05.006
5. Ryan Camilon P, Stokes WA, Nguyen SA, Lentsch EJ (2014) The prognostic significance of age in oropharyngeal squamous cell carcinoma. Oral Oncol 50:431–436. https://doi.org/10.1016/j.oraloncology.2013.12.013
6. Jin LJ, Lamster IB, Greenspan JS, Pitts NB et al (2016) Global burden of oral diseases: emerging concepts, management and interplay with systemic health. Oral Dis 22:609–619. https://doi.org/10.1111/odi.12428
7. Newton JP, Abel EW, Robertson EM, Yemm R (1987) Changes in human masseter and medial pterygoid muscles with age: a study by computed tomography. Gerodontics 3:151–154
8. Liu B, Dion MR, Jurasic MM, Gibson G, Jones JA (2012) Xerostomia and salivary hypofunction in vulnerable elders: prevalence and etiology. Oral Surg Oral Med Oral Pathol Oral Radiol 114:52–60. https://doi.org/10.1016/j.oooo.2011.11.014; [pii]: S2212-4403(12)00035-1
9. Luraschi J, Korgaonkar MS, Whittle T et al (2013) Neuroplasticity in the adaptation to prosthodontic treatment. J Orofac Pain 27:206–216. https://doi.org/10.11607/jop.1097
10. Hartmann R, Müller F (2004) Clinical studies on the appearance of natural anterior teeth in young and old adults. Gerodontology 21:10–16
11. Sheiham A, Steele JG, Marcenes W et al (2001) The relationship among dental status, nutrient intake, and nutritional status in older people. J Dent Res 80:408–413
12. Millwood J, Heath MR (2000) Food choice by older people: the use of semi-structured interviews with open and closed questions. Gerodontology 17:25–32

13. Papas AS, Joshi A, Giunta JL, Palmer CA (1998) Relationships among education, dentate status, and diet in adults. Spec Care Dentist 18:26–32
14. Weiss A, Beloosesky Y, Boaz M et al (2008) Body mass index is inversely related to mortality in elderly subjects. J Gen Intern Med 23:19–24. https://doi.org/10.1007/s11606-007-0429-4
15. Moynihan P (2005) The interrelationship between diet and oral health. Proc Nutr Soc 64:571–580
16. Moynihan PJ, Butler TJ, Thomason JM et al (2000) Nutrient intake in partially dentate patients: the effect of prosthetic rehabilitation. J Dent 28:557–563
17. World Health Organization (2015) World report on ageing and health. WHO Press, Geneva
18. Peltola P, Vehkalahti MM, Wuolijoki-Saaristo K (2004) Oral health and treatment needs of the long-term hospitalised elderly. Gerodontology 21:93–99
19. Bergstrom J (1989) Cigarette smoking as risk factor in chronic periodontal disease. Community Dent Oral Epidemiol 17:245–247
20. Pretty IA, Ellwood RP, Lo EC et al (2014) The Seattle Care Pathway for securing oral health in older patients. Gerodontology 31(Suppl 1):77–87. https://doi.org/10.1111/ger.12098
21. Krall EA, Wehler C, Garcia RI et al (2001) Calcium and vitamin D supplements reduce tooth loss in the elderly. Am J Med 111:452–456
22. Jenson L, Budenz AW, Featherstone JD et al (2007) Clinical protocols for caries management by risk assessment. J Calif Dent Assoc 35:714–723
23. Walls AW, Meurman JH (2012) Approaches to caries prevention and therapy in the elderly. Adv Dent Res 24:36–40. https://doi.org/10.1177/0022034512453590
24. Gunsolley JC (2010) Clinical efficacy of antimicrobial mouthrinses. J Dent 38(Suppl 1):S6–S10. https://doi.org/10.1016/S0300-5712(10)70004-X
25. Sjögren P, Nilsson E, Forsell M et al (2008) A systematic review of the preventive effect of oral hygiene on pneumonia and respiratory tract infection in elderly people in hospitals and nursing homes: effect estimates and methodological quality of randomized controlled trials. J Am Geriatr Soc 56:2124–2130. https://doi.org/10.1111/j.1532-5415.2008.01926.x
26. Sjögren P, Wardh I, Zimmerman M et al (2016) Oral care and mortality in older adults with pneumonia in hospitals or nursing homes: systematic review and meta-analysis. J Am Geriatr Soc 64:2109–2115. https://doi.org/10.1111/jgs.14260
27. Iinuma T, Arai Y, Abe Y et al (2015) Denture wearing during sleep doubles the risk of pneumonia in the very elderly. J Dent Res 94:28S–36S. https://doi.org/10.1177/0022034514552493
28. Stafford GD, Arendorf T, Huggett R (1986) The effect of overnight drying and water immersion on candidal colonization and properties of complete dentures. J Dent 14:52–56
29. Maupome G, Peters D, Rush WA et al (2006) The relationship between cardiovascular xerogenic medication intake and the incidence of crown/root restorations. J Public Health Dent 66:49–56
30. Weeks JC, Dutt A, Robinson PG (2003) Promoting sugar-free medicines: evaluation of a multi-faceted intervention. Community Dent Health 20:246–250
31. Makinen KK, Pemberton D, Cole J et al (1995) Saliva stimulants and the oral health of geriatric patients. Adv Dent Res 9:125–126. https://doi.org/10.1177/08959374950090020901

Malnutrition Unrecognized and Untreated

4

M. Vandewoude and S. Perkisas

Key Messages

- Involuntary weight loss is common in older people and is an unfavorable prognostic sign.
- Health care professionals recognize only part of the malnourished patients as being malnourished, and even fewer malnourished patients classified themselves as being malnourished.
- Three subtypes of malnutrition exist (1) starvation-related without inflammation, (2) chronic disease or conditions that impose sustained mild-to-moderate inflammation (e.g., sarcopenic obesity, organ failure), and (3) acute disease or injury states, when inflammatory response is marked leading to cachexia.
- Most instruments screen for nutritional risk and not for existing malnutrition; this indicates that the first screening level is based on simple measurements. Not all of the screening tools were validated for the old population.
- Only after that a complete nutritional assessment should describe their actual nutritional status.
- Nutritional intervention with optimal dietary patterns should start early.
- Optimal protein intake should be at least 1.2 g/kg/body weight for active older people with an even distribution throughout the day.

M. Vandewoude (✉) · S. Perkisas
University Department Geriatrics, Ziekenhuisnetwerk Antwerpen (ZNA), University of Antwerp, Antwerpen, Belgium
e-mail: maurits.vandewoude@zna.be

J.-P. Michel (ed.), *Prevention of Chronic Diseases and Age-Related Disability*, Practical Issues in Geriatrics, https://doi.org/10.1007/978-3-319-96529-1_4

4.1 Introduction

Life expectancy continues to rise. Many older people are healthy, but others, particularly people of advanced age have several chronic diseases and present with an important comorbidity. Multiple issues associated with aging have an impact on care, including functional impairment, comorbidity, social support, cognitive function, psychological state, and financial stress. Evaluation of the comorbidity in an older person and assessment of the severity of the various pre-existing conditions and their impact on the overall condition are crucial to providing quality care to older individuals. In this respect, a multidisciplinary approach might be useful in the management of the geriatric patient. Although Comprehensive Geriatric Assessment (CGA) should evaluate different domains, malnutrition has a particular place in it because it still is a potentially treatable condition.

4.2 Geriatric Profile

Geriatric patients are not defined by their age but by their general profile. Aging is characterized by loss of organ function such as loss of muscle mass or bone mineral density together with a reduced capability for adapting to changes in the environment (loss of homeostatic mechanisms). These changes in physical function are paralleled by changes in cognitive function, mental health, and socio-economic status. This can lead progressively to a state of increased vulnerability or frailty [1]. This evolution shows a distinct correlation with age. Data from the Belgian Health Surveys 1997–2004 have shown that the percentage of people with frailty as assessed with the VIP-tool (Variable Indicator for Placement) [2] was 5.1% for the people aged 65–70 years, but had already risen to 48.9% in the cohort older than 85 [3]. Further progression of decline in organ function will induce functional impairment and finally disability. Nutritional state is very crucial in this respect. Recent Belgian data from the NutriAction2 surveys show that awareness for malnutrition is not optimal although it is very prevalent with a negative impact on function [4, 5]. Health care professionals recognized only part of the malnourished patients as being malnourished, and even fewer malnourished patients classified themselves as being malnourished. In community dwelling, older people only 43% and in nursing homes 50% of the malnourished patients was recognized by the HCP as such. Only 30% of the malnourished community dwelling older people recognized themselves as malnourished, against only 10% of the malnourished nursing home residents (Fig. 4.1) [5, 6].

4.3 Components of Malnutrition

Involuntary weight loss is common in older people and is an unfavorable prognostic sign. The prevalence of (risk of) malnutrition is high in Belgian older people (≥70 years), especially those living in nursing homes. The NutriAction 2008 study [7] showed that among Belgian older people (≥70 years) living in the community or

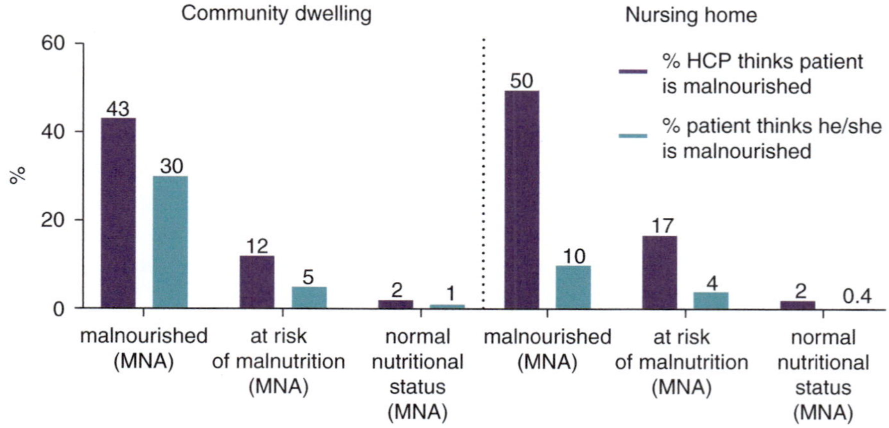

Fig. 4.1 Percentage of health care professionals (HCP) and patients who recognize correctly their nutritional status as well in community dwelling older people as in nursing home residents

in a nursing home, the risk of malnutrition (MNA $\leq$ 11) is highly prevalent (57%), and that 16% was classified as malnourished (BMI < 20 kg/m^2). In 2013, this study was repeated (NutriAction2). The prevalence of malnutrition has remained stable among Belgian older people over the period 2008–2013. The prevalence of the risk of malnutrition (MNA $\leq$11) is 36% in community dwelling older people, and 63% in nursing home residents [4, 5]. Malnutrition remains a major problem, especially for those in nursing homes or with comorbidities such as depression and dementia. The presence of malnutrition and the presence of the risk of malnutrition are different within comorbidities. The highest prevalence occurs in patients with dementia and depression: in community dwelling older people, 14% of the people with dementia is malnourished and 52% is at risk; in the nursing home population 20% is malnourished and 60% is at risk. In community dwelling older people, 17% of the people with depression is malnourished and 47% is at risk; in the nursing home population with depression 22% is malnourished and 52% is at risk.

Historically, malnutrition has been defined as a condition of an imbalance of energy, protein, and other nutrients that cause measurable negative effects on body composition, physical function, and clinical outcomes another definition of malnutrition has been proposed by an International Guideline Consensus Committee, integrating the acuity of the associated disease and inflammation [8]. The committee specified three subtypes of malnutrition using an etiology-based terminology to assist clinicians to make a nutrition diagnosis in clinical practice settings: (1) starvation-related without inflammation, (2) chronic disease or conditions that impose sustained mild-to-moderate inflammation (e.g., sarcopenic obesity, organ failure), and (3) acute disease or injury states, when inflammatory response is marked leading to cachexia.

Starvation is a pure protein-energy deficiency, forcing a reduction in both fat and fat-free mass. The key physiological sign of starvation is that it is reversed solely by the replenishment of nutrients. Age-related decline in muscle mass has been termed sarcopenia, a term first introduced by Rosenberg in 1989 [9]. Since then, the definition of sarcopenia has continued to evolve. The recognition of impairment in muscle strength and functional status with sarcopenia has added the inclusion of function in the definition and therefore in the assessment. So, sarcopenia is defined as the loss of muscle protein mass, muscle strength, and function [10].

In the aging muscle, many changes occur. Some exist at the architectural level, like alterations in muscle composition, or modifications in the characteristics of the muscle fiber itself, where muscle fiber length, orientation, and type may change. Other changes are located at the neuronal level from the central nervous system down to the level of the motor unit and the neuromuscular junction. Also hormonal factors undergo age-related changes that may have an effect on both strength and function. Although many different components are identified, it is still unclear to what degree each of these components contributes to the loss of muscle mass, strength, and function [11].

Severe wasting of both fat and fat-free mass is termed cachexia. Cachexia accompanies diseases such as cancer or immunodeficiency states. Cachexia is best viewed as the cytokine-associated wasting of protein and energy stores due to the effects of disease [12]. Systemic inflammation mediated through cell injury or activation of the immune system triggers an acute inflammatory response. Persons with cachexia lose fat as well as fat-free mass, while maintaining extracellular water and intracellular potassium. The loss of fat-free mass is mainly from the skeletal muscle and is an essential component in the definition. An operational definition of cachexia [12] states that "cachexia, is a complex metabolic syndrome associated with underlying illness and characterized by loss of muscle with or without loss of fat mass. The prominent clinical feature of cachexia is weight loss in adults (corrected for fluid retention)." Other diagnostic criteria for cachexia besides loss of muscle mass and evidence of accelerated protein degradation in muscle are decreased muscle strength, fatigue, anorexia, and biochemical abnormalities characteristic of inflammation, anemia, or hypoalbuminemia. The key clinical question is whether starvation, sarcopenia, and cachexia are distinct entities or represent an interdependent continuum. In the older patient, there can be problems of dietary intake next to the effects of aging per se. On top of this situation, the deleterious effects of existing comorbidities and chronic inflammatory processes are superimposed. When these changes are translated into nutritional concepts, it is clear that in the older patient there is a strong overlap of starvation, sarcopenia, and cachexia. The final result is a complex metabolic state resulting in a therapy resistant malnutrition-sarcopenia syndrome [13].

4.4 Screening Tools

Implementing routine screening to detect malnutrition has been hindered by the lack of universally agreed criteria to identify it. Consequently, there are a variety of nutritional tools in use that incorporate different anthropometric, biochemical, and clinical criteria which have often been developed for use in a particular setting or for a specific patient group. Most instruments screen for nutritional risk and not for existing malnutrition. Actually, this indicates that the first screening level is based on simple measurements that identify people who may be at risk for malnutrition. Only after that a complete nutritional assessment should describe their actual nutritional status with biochemical, anthropometric, functional parameters of muscle strength (handgrip), bio-impedance, and dexa-measurements. Although slight declines in weight have been observed with aging alone, clinically important weight loss (>5% of usual body weight) is almost always the result of disease. In older people, weight loss and low Body Mass Index (BMI, defined as weight in kilograms, divided by height squared) have been associated with adverse outcomes such as decreased functional abilities and increased morbidity and mortality. BMI demonstrates a U-shaped relationship with functional impairment, with greater risk in those with the lowest and highest BMI [14]. The annual incidence of involuntary weight loss (defined as loss of greater than 4% of body weight) was reported to be 13.1% in community-dwelling veterans. Over a 2-year follow-up period, involuntary weight loss was associated with a greater relative risk of mortality (RR = 2.4, 95% confidence interval 1.3–4.4) [15]. Because routine weighing is an inexpensive method to screen for energy undernutrition, patients should be weighed at their primary visit and the weight should be documented in their medical record [16].

The "malnutrition universal screening tool" (MUST) for adults has been developed for multidisciplinary use by the Malnutrition Advisory Group of the British Association for Parenteral and Enteral Nutrition (www.bapen.org.uk) for use in all health care settings. It also has good reproducibility between users and is acceptable to patients and health care workers. The MUST score is able to predict increased mortality in older hospitalized patients [17]. MUST is a five-step screening tool to identify adults, who are malnourished, at risk of undernutrition or obese. It also includes management guidelines which can be used to develop a care plan. The MUST tool scores for Body Mass Index, loss of weight in the past 3–6 months, and the presence of an acute illness or no nutritional intake for 5 days or more.

The NRS (Nutritional Risk Score) [18] is based on the concept that nutritional support is indicated in patients who are severely ill with increased nutritional requirements, or who are severely undernourished, or who have certain degrees of severity of disease in combination with certain degrees of undernutrition. Patients are characterized by scoring the components "undernutrition" and "severity of disease" in four categories (absent, mild, moderate, and severe). The patient can have a score of 0–3 for each component which results in a total score of 0–6. Any patient with a total score ≥3 is considered at nutritional risk. Undernutrition is evaluated using three variables (BMI, percent recent weight loss, and recent change in food intake). The most compromised of the three variables is used to categorize the patient. With age >70 years, a value of 1 is added to the total score.

The SNAQ (Short Nutritional Assessment Questionnaire) was validated in a population of mixed internal, surgical, and oncological patients [19]. It consists of three questions regarding involuntary weight loss, loss of appetite, and recent use of supplemental drinks or tube feeding. Those questions appeared to be the best indicators for malnutrition. The SNAQ has also been validated for an outpatient population [20]. However, it was not specifically validated in an older population.

The Mini Nutritional Assessment (MNA) is both a screening and assessment tool for the identification of malnutrition in older people [21]. The MNA is composed of 18 items, including anthropometric measurements [weight, height, mid-arm circumference, calf circumference, and weight loss during the past 3 months], a global assessment (six questions related to lifestyle, medication, and mobility), a dietary assessment (eight questions related to number of meals, food and fluid intake, and autonomy of feeding), and a subjective assessment (self-perception of health and nutrition). The maximum score is 30 points, with the risk of malnutrition increasing with lower scores. The MNA score was used to classify subjects as well nourished (a score of 24–30), at risk for malnutrition (a score of 17–23.5), or malnourished (a score of <17) according to the original cut-off point of the MNA full test. The screening section of the questionnaire uses 6 items from the global test, namely reduction in food intake, weight loss, mobility, acute stress, neuropsychological problems, and BMI. If the score is 12 points or greater, the patient is not at risk, and there is no need to complete the rest of the questionnaire. If the score is 11 points or less, the patient may be at risk from malnutrition and the full MNA should be completed.

The assessment of nutritional status could be questioned in view of the many non-nutritional factors affecting the results. Subjective assessment of nutritional status has been proposed to overcome these difficulties [22]. Subjective global assessment (SGA) is a validated method of nutritional assessment based on the features of a medical history (weight change, dietary intake change, gastrointestinal symptoms that have persisted for more than 2 weeks, changes in functional capacity) and physical examination (loss of subcutaneous fat, muscle wasting, ankle or sacral edema, and ascites) [23]. The patient-generated-subjective global assessment (PG-SGA) was adapted from the SGA and developed specifically for patients with cancer [24]. It includes additional questions regarding the presence of nutritional symptoms and short-term weight loss. It was designed so that the components of the medical history can be completed by the patient using a check box format. The physical examination is then performed by a health professional, e.g., physician, nurse, or dietitian. The scored PG-SGA is a further development of the PG-SGA concept that incorporates a numerical score as well as providing a global rating of well-nourished, moderately or suspected of being malnourished or severely malnourished. For each component of the scored PG-SGA, points (0–4) are awarded depending on the impact of the symptom on nutritional status. A total score is then summed and this provides a guideline as to the level of nutrition intervention required [25]. The scored PG-SGA, unlike SGA, which is categorical, is a continuous measure. Higher scores indicate a greater risk for malnutrition.

4.5 Nutritional Assessment

Baseline screening for malnutrition is mandatory in the treatment strategy for older patients. As discussed before, several screening instruments have been developed. However, most of them have not been validated in an older population. This is the case for the SNAQ, the MUST, and the NRS although the MUST has shown to be able to predict increased mortality in older hospitalized patients [17]. NRS has proven not sensitive enough to predict weight loss in diseased older subjects [26]. NRS adds one point when age is above 70. In a geriatric population, this item scores 100% positive and therefore has no additional discriminative value.

There is a significant overlap in the methodology of the different screening tools. For example, the assessment of weight loss is a major issue in most of them. Second, the use of BMI is enforced. However, in older people the body length is not a constant factor [27]. It tends to decrease with age. This leads to a systematic error in the calculation and an overestimation of the BMI. Furthermore, in older disabled people body weight and body length are often the result of estimation. The official guidelines for the MUST, for example, give alternative ways for dealing with this problem with the following advice, "If unable to obtain height and weight, see for alternative measurements and use of subjective criteria." When two variables are not measured but estimated, when subsequently one is squared and the quotient is taken, one can doubt the exactness of the final result. On the other hand, when BMI is systematically overrated, a low BMI, indeed, may be a significant sign for the risk of malnutrition. Taking into account the systematic overestimation of BMI, the classical cut-off value of <18.5 [15] may be increased to the cut-off value used in the MUST guideline (<20.0). However, a normal or even high BMI does not exclude nutritional problems. Increase in body fat may, indeed, mimic the loss of muscle mass. It has been corroborated that sarcopenic obesity, or low muscle mass in relation to fat mass, predicted onset of IADL disability in community-dwelling elders who had no disability [28]. In cancer patients, it was shown that sarcopenic obesity was associated with poorer functional status compared with obese patients who did not have sarcopenia and that sarcopenia was an independent predictor of lower survival [29]. This may be particularly important because fat-free mass represents the volume of distribution of many cytotoxic chemotherapy drugs. Estimation of relative sarcopenia (muscle mass adjusted for body fat mass) may, therefore, be a better predictor than absolute sarcopenia.

4.6 Nutritional Management and Intervention

As shown in prevalence studies older adults are at particular risk of sarcopenia, malnutrition, or cachexia [7]. When people get ill, muscle loss occurs early and rapidly. Early intervention is therefore essential in helping to preserve body composition [30].

A first step is the estimation of the energy and protein needs. The energy requirements depend on basal metabolism, physical activity, existing comorbidities, and metabolic stress of acute disease [31]. These requirements may be calculated by predictive equations or measured by indirect calorimetry. However, predictive equations are less accurate for individual patients, whereas indirect calorimetry requires specialized equipment that is not routinely available [32]. The easiest method to estimate energy needs is to use the simple predictive formula that determines daily calorie requirements by multiplying the patient's actual body weight (in kg) by 25–30 kcal [33]. Ideal or adjusted body weight is used for estimating needs of obese and emaciated adults.

Skeletal muscle mass is relatively constant during young- to middle-aged adulthood, suggesting that there is an equilibrium between protein synthesis during absorptive states (i.e., postprandial, following feeding) that is balanced by the catabolism during fasting states. However, this equilibrium in healthy muscle between protein synthesis and breakdown is getting progressively disrupted with aging. In older people, synthesis rate of mixed muscle proteins including myofibrillar and mitochondrial proteins decrease with 30% [34]. Muscle protein synthesis is stimulated by dietary intake of both essential and nonessential amino acids. There is a substantial body of research suggesting that over 80% of the stimulatory effect on protein synthesis observed after a meal can be attributed to amino acids [35]. In older people compared to younger individuals, this stimulatory effect is being blunted but not absent. It can be overruled by increasing the amount of protein. In addition to their role in protein synthesis, amino acids also play a role in the regulation of protein breakdown [36]. Nitrogen balance studies in aging populations (56–80 years of age) have indicated greater protein needs for the elderly (1.14 g/kg/day) relative to the young (0.8 g/kg/day) [37]. This provides critical information in terms of inadequate protein intake as a possible mechanism underlying muscle loss and the development of sarcopenia, particularly because protein intake has been reported as inversely proportional to age. Randomized controlled trial data indicate that it is more important to ingest a sufficient amount of high-quality protein (25–30 g) with each meal rather than 1 large bolus because greater than 30 g in a single meal may not further stimulate muscle protein synthesis [38].

An average daily intake of 1.0–1.2 g protein per kilogram of body weight per day is recommended for older people to maintain and regain lean body mass and function. A higher protein intake (≥1.2 g/kg body weight/day) is advised for those who are exercising and otherwise active. Most older adults who have acute or chronic diseases need even more dietary protein (1.2–1.5 g/kg body weight/day) [39, 40].

Next to the existence of protein-calorie malnutrition attention should be given to specific and selective aspects of malnutrition such as vitamin and mineral deficiencies. Vitamin D has recently received recognition as another potential intervention strategy for sarcopenia. Although our understanding of the relationship between vitamin D and muscle function has advanced over the past decade, a complete understanding of the vitamin D action on muscle tissue and how this translates into improvements in muscular performance are yet to be elucidated. Older adults, however, are at increased risk of developing vitamin D insufficiency and supplementation may be indicated in those older people with low vitamin D levels to combat sarcopenia, functional decline, and falls risk [41].

Overall, preference should be given to nutritional support by adapting a dietary pattern that is adequate in quality in older age to ensure sufficient intakes of protein, vitamin D, antioxidant nutrients, and long-chain polyunsaturated fatty acids. In particular, there is substantial evidence to support the roles of dietary protein and physical activity as key anabolic stimuli for muscle protein synthesis [42]. The addition of oral nutritional supplements or enteral and parenteral feeding might be subsequent steps when calorie or protein requirements cannot be met.

Conclusion

When people grow older, they lose the capacity of adapting well to changes in their environment. This loss of homeostasis in the broad sense leads to an increased vulnerability, called frailty. Although no universal definition has been defined, frailty could be described as an unstable equilibrium carrying a high risk for functional loss. It is a clinical state in which there is an increase in an individual's vulnerability for developing increased dependency and/or mortality when exposed to a stressor [1]. Losing weight with the emergence of malnutrition is part of it. The decline in nutritional status in the geriatric patient is the result of the effects of lower dietary intake (starvation), the effects of aging (sarcopenia), and the effects of acute and chronic inflammatory conditions (cachexia). This results in a complex malnutrition syndrome with a major impact on prognosis and beneficial effects of intended treatment. The screening for comorbidity in older people is essential and nutritional assessment is a major issue in this regard. Difference should be made between assessment of risk and actual nutritional status, which should be assessed with specific malnutrition indices. Body weight assessment with specific attention to unintended weight loss is essential in this evaluation. We should recognize the fact that BMI should be interpreted with caution, but that a low value for BMI still heralds an increased malnutrition risk. Weight loss alone, however, does not identify the full effect of cachexia on physical function. It can be helpful to add to the item of weight loss an estimate of reduction in food intake and systemic inflammation. This would help to identify patients with both adverse function and prognosis. This increased alertness based on a relative subjective global assessment has a lot to offer in the willingness for early intervention. The nutritional assessment must be framed in a larger CGA (comprehensive geriatric assessment) addressing several functional domains. Early intervention with an adequate amount of macronutrients (protein, calories) and micronutrients (vitamins, antioxidants, minerals) offered through a balanced dietary pattern is key in this approach. This may lead to an optimalization of the strategy for the prevention and management of problems in older people.

References

1. Morley JE, Vellas B, van Kan GA et al (2013) Frailty consensus: a call to action. J Am Med Dir Assoc 14:392–397
2. Vandewoude MFJ, Geerts CAM, Paridaens KMJ, D'Hooghe HM (2008) A screening tool for activating liaison geriatrics in general hospitals: the "variable indicative of placement risk" (VIP). Eur J Geriatr 10:120–126
3. Hoeck S, Vandewoude M, Geerts J et al (2007) Déceler la fragilité des Belges de plus de 65 ans vivant à domicile, à l'aide de deux instruments de dépistage. Neuron 12:237–242

4. Van Gossum A, Van Wijngaarden J, Hofstede J et al (2017) Malnutrition is highly prevalent in Belgian nursing home residents and community dwelling older adults, especially in those with depression and dementia. Clin Nutr 36:S67
5. Vandewoude MFJ, van Wijngaarden JP, De Maesschalck L, Luiking YC, Van Gossum A (2018) The prevalence and health burden of malnutrition in Belgian older people in the community or residing in nursing homes: results of the NutriAction II study. Aging Clin Exp Res. https://doi.org/10.1007/s40520-018-0957-2
6. Van Wijngaarden J, Van Gossum A, Rudka T et al (2017) Malnutrition is underestimated by health care professionals in older adults. Clin Nutr 36:S66–S67
7. Vandewoude M, Van Gossum A (2013) Nutritional screening strategy in nonagenarians: the value of the MNA-SF (mini nutritional assessment short form) in NutriAction. J Nutr Health Aging 17:310–314
8. Jensen GL, Mirtallo J, Compher C et al (2010) Adult starvation and disease-related malnutrition: a proposal for etiology-based diagnosis in the clinical practice setting from the International Consensus Guideline Committee. Clin Nutr 29:151–153
9. Rosenberg I (1989) Summary comments. Am J Clin Nutr 50:1231–1233
10. Cruz-Jentoft AJ, Baeyens JP, Bauer JM et al (2010) Sarcopenia: European consensus on definition and diagnosis: report of the European Working Group on Sarcopenia in Older People. Age Ageing 39:412–423
11. Perkisas S, De Cock A, Verhoeven V, Vandewoude M (2016) Physiological and architectural changes in the ageing muscle and their relation to strength and function in sarcopenia. Eur Geriatr Med 7:201–206. https://doi.org/10.1016/j.eurger.2015.12.016
12. Evans WJ, Morley JE, Argiles J et al (2008) Cachexia: a new definition. Clin Nutr 27:793–799
13. Vandewoude MF, Alish CJ, Sauer AC et al (2012) Malnutrition-sarcopenia syndrome: is this the future of nutrition screening and assessment for older adults? J Aging Res 2012:651570
14. Vandewoude M, Hoeck S, Geerts J et al (2008) Mobility and frailty in community-dwelling older people: the effect of weight loss. J Nutr Health Aging 12:573
15. Flegal KM, Graubard BI, Williamson DF et al (2005) Excess deaths associated with underweight, overweight, and obesity. JAMA 293:1861–1867
16. Reuben DB (2007) Quality indicators for the care of undernutrition in vulnerable elders. J Am Geriatr Soc 55(Suppl 2):S438–S442
17. Henderson S, Moore N, Lee E et al (2008) Do the malnutrition universal screening tool (MUST) and Birmingham nutrition risk (BNR) score predict mortality in older hospitalised patients? BMC Geriatr 8:26
18. Kondrup J, Rasmussen HH, Hamberg O et al (2003) Nutritional risk screening (NRS 2002): a new method based on an analysis of controlled clinical trials. Clin Nutr 22:321–336
19. Kruizenga HM, Seidell JC, de Vet HC et al (2005) Development and validation of a hospital screening tool for malnutrition: the short nutritional assessment questionnaire (SNAQ). Clin Nutr 24:75–82
20. Neelemaat F, Kruizenga HM, de Vet HC et al (2008) Screening malnutrition in hospital outpatients. Can the SNAQ malnutrition screening tool also be applied to this population? Clin Nutr 27:439–446
21. Guigoz Y, Vellas B, Garry P (1994) Mini nutritional assessment: a practical assessment tool for grading the nutritional state of elderly patients. Facts Res Gerontol 4:15–59
22. Jeejeebhoy KN, Detsky AS, Baker JP (1990) Assessment of nutritional status. JPEN J Parenter Enteral Nutr 14:193S–196S
23. Detsky AS, McLaughlin JR, Baker JP et al (1987) What is subjective global assessment of nutritional status? JPEN J Parenter Enteral Nutr 11:8–13
24. Ottery FD (1994) Rethinking nutritional support of the cancer patient: the new field of nutritional oncology. Semin Oncol 21:770–778
25. Ottery F (2000) Patient-generated subjective global assessment. In: PD MC, Polisena CG (eds) The clinical guide to oncology nutrition. American Dietetic Association, Chicago, IL, pp 11–23

26. Ritz P, Prod'Homme F, Berger V et al (2007) Nutritional risk score is not sensitive enough to predict weight loss in diseased elderly subjects. J Nutr Health Aging 11:389–392
27. Van Hoeyweghen RJ, De Leeuw IH, Vandewoude MF (1992) Creatinine arm index as alternative for creatinine height index. Am J Clin Nutr 56:611–615
28. Baumgartner RN, Wayne SJ, Waters DL et al (2004) Sarcopenic obesity predicts instrumental activities of daily living disability in the elderly. Obes Res 12:1995–2004
29. Prado CM, Lieffers JR, McCargar LJ et al (2008) Prevalence and clinical implications of sarcopenic obesity in patients with solid tumours of the respiratory and gastrointestinal tracts: a population-based study. Lancet Oncol 9:629–635
30. Vandewoude M, Bautmans I (2012) Sarcopenia: is it preventable? In: Cruz-Jentoft A, Morley J (eds) Sarcopenia. Wiley/Blackwell, West Sussex, pp 324–337
31. Correia MI, Hegazi RA, Higashiguchi T et al (2014) Evidence-based recommendations for addressing malnutrition in health care: an updated strategy from the feedM.E. Global Study Group. J Am Med Dir Assoc 15:544–550
32. Trevino-Aguirre E, Lopez-Teros T, Gutierrez-Robledo L et al (2014) Availability and use of dual energy X-ray absorptiometry (DXA) and bio-impedance analysis (BIA) for the evaluation of sarcopenia by Belgian and Latin American geriatricians. J Cachexia Sarcopenia Muscle 5:79–81
33. McClave SA, Martindale RG, Vanek VW et al (2009) Guidelines for the provision and assessment of nutrition support therapy in the adult critically ill patient: Society of Critical Care Medicine (SCCM) and American Society for Parenteral and Enteral Nutrition (A.S.P.E.N.). JPEN J Parenter Enteral Nutr 33:277–316
34. Volpi E, Rasmussen BB (2000) Nutrition and muscle protein metabolism in the elderly. Diabetes Nutr Metab 13:99–107
35. Volpi E, Kobayashi H, Sheffield-Moore M et al (2003) Essential amino acids are primarily responsible for the amino acid stimulation of muscle protein anabolism in healthy elderly adults. Am J Clin Nutr 78:250–258
36. Zanchi NE, Nicastro H, Lancha AH Jr (2008) Potential antiproteolytic effects of L-leucine: observations of in vitro and in vivo studies. Nutr Metab (Lond) 5:20
37. Campbell WW, Crim MC, Dallal GE et al (1994) Increased protein requirements in elderly people: new data and retrospective reassessments. Am J Clin Nutr 60:501–509
38. Symons TB, Sheffield-Moore M, Wolfe RR et al (2009) A moderate serving of high-quality protein maximally stimulates skeletal muscle protein synthesis in young and elderly subjects. J Am Diet Assoc 109:1582–1586
39. Bauer J, Biolo G, Cederholm T et al (2013) Evidence-based recommendations for optimal dietary protein intake in older people: a position paper from the PROT-AGE Study Group. JAm Med Dir Assoc 14:542–559
40. Deutz NE, Bauer JM, Barazzoni R et al (2014) Protein intake and exercise for optimal muscle function with aging: recommendations from the ESPEN Expert Group. Clin Nutr 33:929–936
41. Dawson-Hughes B (2008) Serum 25-hydroxyvitamin D and functional outcomes in the elderly. Am J Clin Nutr 88:537S–540S
42. Robinson SM, Reginster JY, Rizzoli R et al (2018) Does nutrition play a role in the prevention and management of sarcopenia? Clin Nutr 37(4):1121–1132

Sarcopenia: Preventable and Reversible

5

Alfonso J. Cruz-Jentoft

Key Messages

- Sarcopenia is associated with many undesirable outcomes: mortality, functional decline, falls and fractures, hospital admission and reduced quality of life.
- It is more frequent with increasing age, female gender, low protein intake, low levels of physical activity, not engaging in regular exercise and other habits.
- Adding resistance exercise to usual aerobic exercise is key in preventing sarcopenia. Comprehensive resistance exercise programs are needed to treat this condition, when present.
- A healthy diet that increases the amount of proteins is also important to prevent sarcopenia from a lifelong perspective. When sarcopenia is present, proper nutritional intervention—frequently with the use of oral nutrition supplements—is needed to improve muscle function.

5.1 What Is Sarcopenia?

Sarcopenia is a progressive and generalized loss of skeletal muscle mass and function that increases the risk of adverse outcomes in old age [1].

The term sarcopenia is quite recent in the medical literature. It was proposed in 1998, and derives from two Greek words: *sarx* for flesh and *penia* for loss to describe a well-known long-standing observation: the progressive muscle wasting that many individuals show when aging, that is commonly associated with reduced muscle strength and power, and affects mobility and functional independence [2].

Initially, sarcopenia was approached by focusing on the loss of muscle mass that starts in adult age, but increasing evidence showed that measured muscle mass was

A. J. Cruz-Jentoft
Hospital Universitario Ramón y Cajal (IRYCS), Madrid, Spain
e-mail: alfonsojose.cruz@salud.madrid.org

J.-P. Michel (ed.), *Prevention of Chronic Diseases and Age-Related Disability*, Practical Issues in Geriatrics, https://doi.org/10.1007/978-3-319-96529-1_5

only weakly associated with mobility problems and disability, so interest gradually switched to muscle function. In 2010, several international groups proposed consensus definitions that incorporated muscle strength and physical performance to the concept of sarcopenia [3]. The most widely used is the definition of the European Working Group for Sarcopenia in Older People (EWGSOP), that defines sarcopenia as the association of a reduced muscle mass with a reduced muscle strength or physical performance (or both) [1]. Only in 2016, the US version of the International Classification of Diseases (ICD-10) coded sarcopenia as a specific disease.

Sarcopenia can be best understood as an organ failure (skeletal muscle insufficiency), contrasting with frailty, that is considered a whole-body issue (see next chapter) [4]. Sarcopenia usually presents as a slowly progressive, age-associated chronic disorder, but can also develop acutely (i.e., during hospital admission or acute immobility), so considering sarcopenia as a chronic or acute skeletal muscle insufficiency may be an accurate clinical paradigm, already in use for other organs or systems (i.e., renal or cardiac insufficiency).

5.2 Why Is Sarcopenia a Problem?

Epidemiological studies have shown that sarcopenia is common in old age, it's prevalence rising with increasing age. However, published prevalence and incidence rates are quite variable, depending on the population age, gender, and characteristics, the use of different measures of muscle mass and function, and the choice of cutoff points [5]. Reported prevalence in community dwelling older people ranges from 1 to 33%, most recent epidemiological reports seem to be in the 15–20% range. Prevalence is higher in nursing homes or long-term care settings, and also in older people admitted to the hospital. This means that at least one in five older individuals may suffer from sarcopenia.

Sarcopenia is associated with many undesirable outcomes. Sarcopenic individuals have a higher mortality (at least threefold), high risk of functional decline and fall more frequently. It also seems to be associated with a higher risk of hospital admission and may be linked to longer stays and a higher risk of fractures [6]. It also carries a reduced quality of life that has prompted the development of specific instruments [7]. Moreover, sarcopenia is a real public health burden [8], and recent evidence links sarcopenia with increased health care costs [9]. Costs associated with increased disability have not been properly studied.

5.3 Life Course Perspective and Determinants of Sarcopenia

Sarcopenia does not come from clear sky, it develops along the lifetime of an individual, starting very early in life. Weight at birth has been shown to be a determinant of sarcopenia, probably through its influence on peak muscle mass and strength in early adulthood [10]. Little is known about how very early interventions may have an impact in late life sarcopenia.

Recent research has focused on the determinants of sarcopenia in adulthood. Some of them are well established: increasing age, female gender, body frame, ethnicity, and heritability have been confirmed in different studies. However, these determinants cannot be changed. More important from a preventive point of view, lower food intake, reduced protein intake, malnutrition, low levels of physical activity, and not engaging in regular exercise are all risk factors of sarcopenia, while healthy food patterns and having appropriate levels of vitamin D seem to be protective [11]. Some diseases (diabetes mellitus, osteoporosis, osteoarthritis, and a number of other comorbid diseases) and multimorbidity by itself also increase the risk of sarcopenia. New risk factors, as poor sleep or pain, may also have a role. All these risk factors seem to be cumulative.

Individuals who become sarcopenic and have a negative lifestyle or some comorbid diseases may have an accelerated course of the disease. Sarcopenia reduces physical activity—by reducing mobility—, increases nutrient needs, and may have an impact on comorbid diseases (for instance, modifying the effect of drugs through changes in body composition). Thus, when managing sarcopenic individuals, tertiary prevention of existing risk factors is still needed.

5.4 Preventing Sarcopenia

Being sarcopenia a recently identified clinical problem, no long-term prevention trials in large populations have been yet performed. However, epidemiological studies and some small prevention studies may offer some guidelines.

Resistance exercise seems to be a key in preventing sarcopenia. It is quite clear that physical exercise has a positive impact on muscle mass and muscle function in healthy subjects aged 60 years and older [12]. Exercise improves physical performance (chair rising, gait speed, balance), even when no changes in muscle mass are shown. Thus, adding resistance exercise to the usual recommendation to do aerobic exercise may have a role in preventing sarcopenia. This should start early in life, as muscle mass and function loss starts early in adulthood and is more prominent after 50 years old. The role of aerobic or balance exercise in preventing sarcopenia. Increasing daily physical activity seems also advisable although the effect or size of such increase is yet undetermined.

The other cornerstone of sarcopenia prevention is diet. Healthier dietary habits, especially those that ensure an appropriate amount of proteins and avoid vitamin D deficiencies, will probably prevent sarcopenia—and other chronic diseases [13, 14]. Protein intake seems to be particularly important. In fact, the former recommendation of a minimum intake of 0.8 g of protein per kg of body weight and day for adults has recently been increased by some international organizations to a minimum of 1.0–1.2 g for older adults to prevent sarcopenia and frailty [15, 16]. Thus, a recommendation to increase protein intake seems sound advice to prevent sarcopenia. Some data also suggest that the combination of exercise and diet may have a synergistic effect [17].

Of course, preventive measures that need changes in lifestyle that have been present for 40–50 years are specially challenging, and many barriers have been found (education, poverty, costs and availability of exercise programs, psychological barriers, and others), but prevention of sarcopenia is key in the societies' quest to prevent physical disability in old age.

Although some persons may consider the use of botanicals or alternative medicine approaches to prevent sarcopenia, there is no evidence to date that this approach has any significant effect [18].

5.5 Reversing Sarcopenia

More information is available on the treatment of sarcopenia. It is now clear that sarcopenia is not a permanent state, and it can be reversed, either spontaneously (i.e., acute sarcopenia after an acute condition is cured) or by interventions.

Management of sarcopenia starts with the identification and management of any underlying cause found by a comprehensive geriatric assessment. Nutrition and physical exercise are the cornerstones of treatment [12]. No drug has yet been approved for this condition although many are in development [19], some even in phase 2 trials [20].

Again, resistance exercise is the first and most important treatment to reverse sarcopenia. It has to be prescribed properly and adapted to the needs of each individual. Total body exercise routines that include routines for major muscle groups, for 30–60 min three to four times a week, using multi-joint approaches with exercise machines at an intensity of 65–75% of the maximum have the best evidence [21]. Adding aerobic exercise training may also benefit skeletal muscle and improve insulin sensitivity. Exercise has to be properly prescribed by a physician or physical therapist and is most probably beneficial when properly supervised and sustained a long time.

Correction of nutritional deficits is also needed in sarcopenic patients [22]. Caloric intake should be increased to cover increased demands posed by exercise. Protein requirements may be increased, when sarcopenia is present, to the range of 1.2–1.5 g of protein per kilogram of body weight and day, with the only exception of subjects with stage 4 or 5 renal failure [15]. Essential amino acids (EAA) supplements including around 2.5 g of leucine and β-hydroxy β-methylbutyric acid (HMB) supplements may also help to improve muscle mass and function parameters [5]. Correction of vitamin D deficiencies is needed for proper muscle function, but the role of vitamin D when blood levels are normal it is yet to be determined. When requirements cannot be reached by modifying usual diet, oral nutritional supplements are needed to meet these needs. Supplements should be used for at least 3 months to be most effective.

References

1. Cruz-Jentoft AJ, Baeyens JP, Bauer JM, Boirie Y, Cederholm T, Landi F et al (2010) Sarcopenia: European consensus on definition and diagnosis: report of the European Working Group on sarcopenia in older people. Age Ageing 39(4):412–423
2. Rosenberg IH (1997) Sarcopenia: origins and clinical relevance. J Nutr 127(5 Suppl):990S–991S
3. Morley JE, Cruz-Jentoft AJ (2012) Definitions of sarcopenia. In: Cruz-Jentoft AJ, Morley JE (eds) Sarcopenia. Wiley-Blackwell, Hoboken, NJ, pp 8–19
4. Cruz-Jentoft AJ (2016) Sarcopenia, the last organ insufficiency. Eur Geriatr Med 7(3): 195–196
5. Cruz-Jentoft AJ, Landi F, Schneider SM, Zuniga C, Arai H, Boirie Y et al (2014) Prevalence of and interventions for sarcopenia in ageing adults: a systematic review. Report of the International Sarcopenia Initiative (EWGSOP and IWGS). Age Ageing 43(6):748–759
6. Beaudart C, Zaaria M, Pasleau F, Reginster J-Y, Bruyère O (2017) Health outcomes of sarcopenia: a systematic review and meta-analysis. PLoS One 12(1):e0169548
7. Beaudart C, Reginster J-Y, Geerinck A, Locquet M, Bruyère O (2017) Current review of the SarQoL®: a health-related quality of life questionnaire specific to sarcopenia. Expert Rev Pharmacoecon Outcomes Res 17(4):335–341
8. Ethgen O, Beaudart C, Buckinx F, Bruyère O, Reginster JY (2017) The future prevalence of sarcopenia in Europe: a claim for public health action. Calcif Tissue Int 100(3):229–234
9. Antunes AC, Araújo DA, Veríssimo MT, Amaral TF (2017) Sarcopenia and hospitalisation costs in older adults: a cross-sectional study. Nutr Diet J Dietit Assoc Aust 74(1):46–50
10. Sayer AA, Syddall H, Martin H, Patel H, Baylis D, Cooper C (2008) The developmental origins of sarcopenia. J Nutr Health Aging 12(7):427–432
11. Shaw SC, Dennison EM, Cooper C (2017) Epidemiology of sarcopenia: determinants throughout the Lifecourse. Calcif Tissue Int 101(3):229–247
12. Beaudart C, Dawson A, Shaw SC, Harvey NC, Kanis JA, Binkley N et al (2017) Nutrition and physical activity in the prevention and treatment of sarcopenia: systematic review. Osteoporos Int 28(6):1817–1833
13. Robinson SM, Reginster JY, Rizzoli R, Shaw SC, Kanis JA, Bautmans I et al (2017) Does nutrition play a role in the prevention and management of sarcopenia? Clin Nutr 37(4):1121–1132. https://doi.org/10.1016/j.clnu.2017.08.016 [Epub ahead of print]
14. Naseeb MA, Volpe SL (2017) Protein and exercise in the prevention of sarcopenia and aging. Nutr Res 40:1–20
15. Bauer J, Biolo G, Cederholm T, Cesari M, Cruz-Jentoft AJ, Morley JE et al (2013) Evidence-based recommendations for optimal dietary protein intake in older people: a position paper from the PROT-AGE Study Group. J Am Med Dir Assoc 14(8):542–559
16. Deutz NEP, Bauer JM, Barazzoni R, Biolo G, Boirie Y, Bosy-Westphal A et al (2014) Protein intake and exercise for optimal muscle function with aging: recommendations from the ESPEN Expert Group. Clin Nutr 33(6):929–936
17. Denison HJ, Cooper C, Sayer AA, Robinson SM (2015) Prevention and optimal management of sarcopenia: a review of combined exercise and nutrition interventions to improve muscle outcomes in older people. Clin Interv Aging 10:859–869
18. Rondanelli M, Miccono A, Peroni G, Guerriero F, Morazzoni P, Riva A et al (2016) A systematic review on the effects of botanicals on skeletal muscle health in order to prevent sarcopenia. Evid Based Complement Alternat Med 2016:5970367
19. Morley JE (2016) Pharmacologic options for the treatment of sarcopenia. Calcif Tissue Int 98(4):319–333

20. Rooks D, Praestgaard J, Hariry S, Laurent D, Petricoul O, Perry RG et al (2017) Treatment of sarcopenia with Bimagrumab: results from a phase II, randomized, controlled, proof-of-concept study. J Am Geriatr Soc 65(9):1988–1995
21. Law TD, Clark LA, Clark BC (2016) Resistance exercise to prevent and manage sarcopenia and dynapenia. Annu Rev Gerontol Geriatr 36(1):205–228
22. Malafarina V, Uriz-Otano F, Iniesta R, Gil-Guerrero L (2013) Effectiveness of nutritional supplementation on muscle mass in treatment of sarcopenia in old age: a systematic review. J Am Med Dir Assoc 14(1):10–17

6 Frailty Is Not a Fatality

Elisa Zengarini and Antonio Cherubini

Key Messages

- Frailty corresponds to an extreme vulnerability to poor resolution of homeostasis after stressors, due to loss of physiological reserve across multiple systems, which causes an increased risk of adverse health-related outcomes.
- The prevalence of frailty is higher in women and increases with age although the signs and symptoms of frailty are not rare in the middle-aged population.
- Frailty is a dynamic process; the recognition and modification of pre-clinical manifestations and modifiable risk factors, also among adults and young individuals is essential.
- Since frailty is a public health priority, its assessment should be integrated into routine clinical practice for older patients, encouraging the early identification of at-risk individuals and subsequent interventions.
- Frailty and pre-frailty are potentially reversible. Solid evidence supports the efficacy of physical exercise. Current evidence supporting nutrition interventions is scare. Multicomponent interventions, after a global geriatric assessment, appears the best way of reversing the frailty process.

6.1 Definition

Frailty is a condition of extreme vulnerability to poor resolution of homeostasis after stressors, due to loss of physiological reserve across multiple systems, which causes an increased risk of adverse health-related outcomes [1, 2]. Frail older adults

E. Zengarini · A. Cherubini (✉)
Geriatria, Accettazione geriatrica e Centro di ricerca per l'invecchiamento, IRCCS-INRCA, Ancona, Italy
e-mail: a.cherubini@inrca.it

J.-P. Michel (ed.), *Prevention of Chronic Diseases and Age-Related Disability*, Practical Issues in Geriatrics, https://doi.org/10.1007/978-3-319-96529-1_6

have higher risk of adverse health events, including falls, delirium, disability onset, hospitalization, institutionalization, and death [1–3].

6.2 Frailty Identification and Assessment

Although the definition of frailty is agreed on, there is not currently a universally accepted set of criteria to diagnose frailty. Different models have been developed to operationalize frailty diagnosis in research settings and clinical practice. Among them, the phenotype model [1] and the accumulation of deficits model [4] are those most commonly used. In the Cardiovascular Health Study, Fried validated the frailty phenotype using five criteria: unintentional weight loss, self-reported exhaustion, weak grip strength, slow gait speed, low physical activity. Frailty was defined as a clinical syndrome characterized by the presence of three or more criteria, while pre-frailty was identified by the presence of one or two criteria [1].

At variance, the Frailty Index developed by Rockwood in the Canadian Study of Health and Aging is a mathematical construct to measure the cumulative accumulation of deficits (e.g., symptoms, signs, disabilities, diseases, and laboratory abnormalities) over time [4]. It is calculated as a ratio between the number of deficits observed in the individual divided by the total number of deficit considered. Although originally developed using 92 variables [4], shorter versions of the Frailty Index considering no more than 20 deficits have also been validated [5].

A recent review found 67 different set of criteria to identify frailty [6]. The most common purposes of the instruments were to assess frailty as risk factor for adverse health outcomes (31.3%) and identify risk factor for frailty (22.3%), while few studies used frailty as a guide for clinical decision-making (2.3%) and as a target for intervention (2.3%).

Several instruments demonstrated predictive validity for the risk of adverse health outcomes in different cohorts of older subjects. However, they are built on distinctive concepts of frailty and when compared each other, they identify different older adults as frail [7]. For instance, the FRAIL questionnaire based on five self-reported criteria is suited for clinical screening [8]. The Gérontopôle Frailty Screening Tool (GFST) has been developed to increase awareness of frailty among general practitioners and facilitate screening in primary care [9]. On the other hand, the Frailty index derived from Comprehensive Geriatric Assessment (FI-CGA) is designed for frailty assessment in the clinical setting [10]. Also physical performance measures (e.g., gait speed, the short physical performance battery) have been studied as suitable tools for the assessment of frailty [11]. They are reliable, not time-consuming, objective, and repeatable in the same subject over time and thus they may be easily included in the routine medical examination. In a recent international survey, the most commonly used measure to assess frailty was gait speed test [12].

6.3 Epidemiology

In a systematic review based on 21 cohorts involving 61,500 participants, 10.7% of community-dwelling older persons were identified as frail and another 41.6% as prefrail. However, the prevalence of frailty varies considerably (range 4.0–59.1%) because of different definitions and inclusion criteria adopted among different studies [13]. The prevalence is higher in women and increases with age although the signs and symptoms of frailty are not rare in the middle-aged population [14]. Data from the Survey of Health, Aging and Retirement in Europe (SHARE) showed that among European individuals 50–65 years of age, 4.1% were frail, and 37.4% were prefrail, while in the 65 years and older group 17% were frail and 42.3% prefrail. The frailty criteria more commonly reported in the middle-aged group were exhaustion and low activity, while exhaustion, weakness, slowness, and low activity were frequent in the 65 years and older group [14]. Moreover, frailty is consistently associated with some ethnic groups, e.g., black and Hispanic, living in residential care and lower education and poverty [1, 13–15].

6.4 The Course of Frailty and Its Implications

The pathophysiological pathways underlying the development of frailty are not yet clearly identified. Frailty is the result of an accelerated and cumulative decline across multiple systems (i.e., the skeletal and muscular system, the brain, the immune, inflammatory, and endocrine system). Several theories of frailty have been proposed. Fried et al. conceptualized frailty as a geriatric syndrome, describing a vicious cycle where multiple risk factors and conditions are interacting not only to cause frailty but also to promote its progression [1]. On the other hand, Rockwood et al. proposed a stochastic model where deficit accumulation results from interactions between two processes: on one side, environmental stresses, causing damage, and on the other the systems that control damage and recovery time. The exponential increase in the number of health deficits with age corresponds to the exponential increase of recovery time [16].

In any case, frailty is not a static condition, but instead a dynamic process. In the literature, different studies investigated the natural history of frailty and the determinants of the transition between different stages of frailty over time. In a prospective cohort study of 754 predominantly European American community-living persons, Gill showed that frailty is a dynamic process with frequent transitions between frailty states over time: 57% of participants has at least one transition over 4.5 years. Specifically, transitions to states of greater frailty were more common (43%) than transitions to states of milder frailty (23%), while the probability of transitioning from being frail to nonfrail was very low (0–0.9%) [17]. Rockwood analyzed data for community-dwelling subjects (age 15–102 years at baseline) in the longitudinal component of the National Population Health Survey with seven 2-year cycles to estimate the outcomes of frailty measured in terms of Frailty Index. In this study, the scale has been divided into different categories: relatively fit (Frailty Index ≤0.03, i.e., no or only one deficit), less fit (0.03 < Frailty Index ≤0.10), least fit (0.10 < Frailty Index ≤0.21), frail (Frailty Index >0.21), and most frail (Frailty Index ≥0.45). At all ages, the 160-month mortality rate was lower among relatively fit people than among those who were frail (e.g., 2% vs. 16% at age 40; 42% vs. 83% at age 75 or older). Moreover, they demonstrated that the relatively fittest people at baseline tended to remain healthy, while the chance of complete recovery declined with age. The chance of staying at the highest level of fitness across all seven cycles declined with age, while the chance of becoming frail increased [3]. In a study of frailty transitions among participants in the San Antonio Longitudinal Study of Aging (SALSA) cohort, diabetes with macrovascular complications, lower education, and longer follow-up intervals were predictors of frailty worsening [18]. Shardell demonstrated that prefrail participants with lower 25-hydroxyvitamin D were 8.9% more likely to die, 3% more likely to transition to frailty, and 7.7% less likely to become robust. On the other hand, transitions from robustness or frailty were not associated with serum 25-hydroxyvitamin D [19]. Lee et al. examined the natural history of transition between frailty states in a cohort of community-living older Chinese people. Among prefrail subjects, a quarter of both genders recovered into the robust state, while 11.1% of men and 6.6% of women worsened into frailty. Moreover, they found significant factors associated with worsening or less improvement in transition between frailty states (older age, history of stroke, lower cognitive functions, diabetes, osteoarthritis, cancer, lung disease, hospitalizations), while higher socioeconomic status was protective [20]. Recently, Pollack and colleagues in a perspective cohort study of 5086 community-dwelling men found that over 4.6 years 35% progressed in frailty status or died, 15% improved, but only 0.5% of them from frail to robust. A comprehensive evaluation of potential determinants of transition in frailty status showed that factors associated with improvement in frailty status included greater leg power, being married, good or excellent self-reported health. On the other hand, any instrumental activity of daily living (IADL) limitations, low albumin levels, high interleukin-6 levels, and presence of chronic obstructive pulmonary disease or diabetes mellitus were associated with lower likelihood of improvement in frailty status [21].

These evidence suggest that frailty is potentially reversible, particularly in the early stages. It would be extremely important to know the life expectancy of older subjects with frailty, but there is currently no study that can provide this information. A better understanding and management of modifiable clinical, social, and functional risk factors may increase the recovery rate of the prefrail individuals or prevent their progression to frailty. Given its multidomain nature, a comprehensive approach is necessary to target frailty and associated factors. Because the improvement in frailty status has been associated with social, functional, and clinical factors, effective strategies may include rehabilitation and interventions that target strength and lower extremity power, social support, nutritional interventions, and improvement management of comorbidity [21].

In the World Report on Ageing and Health published by the World Health Organization, frailty has been considered as a progressive decline in physiological systems that results in decreased *intrinsic capacity*. The intrinsic capacity is defined as the composite of all the physical and mental (including psychosocial) capacities of an individual. The combination of intrinsic capacity with relevant environmental characteristics and their interactions defines the *functional ability* of the individual. The report defines healthy aging as the process of developing and maintaining the functional ability that enables well-being in older age. Thus, healthy aging reflects the interactions between individuals and the environments, resulting in trajectories of both intrinsic capacity and functional ability [22]. It is noticeable that the prevention of frailty as well as an effective promotion of healthy aging should adopt a life-course perspective. The functional status at older age is the result of behaviors and conditions occurring in the individual during the entire life and the interaction with the environment.

6.5 Interventions

Frailty is a public health priority [23]. Multiple interventions targeting frailty have been investigated. Solid evidence supports the efficacy of exercise in frail older people. A high-intensity progressive resistance training of the hip and knee extensor (chosen because of their importance in functional activities) improved muscle strength and size with associated improvement in mobility and level of physical activity in frail older nursing home residents [24]. Moreover, Gill showed that a program targeting underlying impairments in physical abilities (e.g., balance, muscle strength, ability to transfer from one position to another, and mobility) reduced the progression of functional decline also among physically frail elderly persons living at home [25]. In a more recent trial, the Lifestyle Interventions and Independence for Elders pilot (LIFE-P) study, the incidence of major mobility disability over 2.6 years was reduced in the exercise group compared with a successful aging educational program group. The physical activity program consisted of a combination of walking at moderate intensity, resistance exercises, balance, stretching, and behavioral counseling [26]. Further analyses from the LIFE-P study explored the effects of physical activity on frailty status. Cesari et al. showed that after 12 months of follow-up regular physical activity reduced the frailty prevalence. Moreover, in comparison to successful aging participants, the mean number of frailty criteria in the physical activity group was notably reduced, especially for at-risk individuals (i.e., participants with frailty, and those with multimorbidity) [27]. Exercise has a positive impact on physical determinants and functional outcomes, even if the most effective type and intensity of exercise is uncertain. However, multicomponent training interventions (i.e., focusing on resistance, balance, aerobic, and flexibility training), of long duration (≥5 months), performed three times per week, for 30–45 min per session, generally had superior outcomes than other exercise programs [28].

Although individual nutritional status as well as the dietary style and nutrient intake (e.g., vitamin D) have been demonstrated associated with frailty, current evidence supporting the efficacy of nutritional interventions is scanty [24].

A recent review using the level of frailty as intervention target selected 14 studies designed to prevent or reduce the level of frailty among community-dwelling older adults. The interventions included physical activity, physical activity combined with nutrition or with nutrition and memory training, home modifications, prehabilitation (physical therapy plus exercise plus home modifications), and Comprehensive Geriatric Assessment (CGA). Particularly, the physical activity intervention mostly included strength, balance, coordination, flexibility, and aerobic exercises provided by exercise professionals, with sessions ranging in frequency from once weekly to 5 days per week. Nine of the 14 studies reported that the intervention reduced the level of frailty. On the other hand, studies using Comprehensive Geriatric Assessment had mixed findings [29]. Nevertheless, currently implications of change in frailty level on clinical outcome are not well known. Frost recently evaluated the effectiveness of home- and community-based health promotion interventions on functioning and frailty in individuals with mild or pre-frailty. They identified seven trials: six studies evaluating exercise intervention (single intervention or two intervention, i.e., two exercise interventions or exercise plus nutritions) and one study telemonitoring. Group exercise interventions showed positive effects on functioning, but these were mixed and based on small, low quality studies [30].

In current clinical practice, the gold standard for the management of frailty is the Comprehensive Geriatric Assessment (CGA). The CGA is a multidisciplinary diagnostic process intended to determine a frail elderly person's medical, psychosocial, and functional capabilities and limitations in order to develop a personalized intervention of care and follow-up. This approach is sensitive to detection of levels of frailty [10]. Moreover, this process is closely linked to interventions with subsequent relevant outcomes. Several evidences showed as CGA improves health-related outcomes in frail patients in different setting as hospital [31], home care [32], and nursing home [33].

The relevance of prevention and management of frailty has been recognized by international bodies. The European Commission has recently created the European Scaling-up Strategy in Active and Healthy Ageing including an action group focused on the prevention of frailty and functional (both cognitive and physical) decline [29]. Another relevant European project founded by the Innovative Medicines Initiatives is the Sarcopenia and Physical fRailty IN older people: multi-componenT Treatment strategies (SPRINTT) Study, a large clinical trial specifically designed to implement frailty care and prevention across Europe. In SPRINTT, the efficacy of a multicomponent intervention, based on long-term structured physical activity (including aerobic, strength, flexibility, and balance training), nutritional counseling/dietary intervention, and an information and communication technology intervention, for preventing mobility disability is tested in comparison with a healthy aging lifestyle education program in community-dwelling older persons with physical frailty and sarcopenia [34, 35].

Conclusion

As the world's population ages, the prevention and management of frailty should take on primary relevance. Frailty assessment should be integrated into routine clinical practice for older patients, encouraging the early identification of at-risk individuals and subsequent interventions. Future studies should focus on trajectories of frailty, and thus on the recognition and modification of pre-clinical manifestations and modifiable risk factors, also among adults and young individuals, evaluating complex multicomponent interventions.

References

1. Fried LP, Tangen CM, Walston J et al (2001) Frailty in older adults: evidence for a phenotype. J Gerontol A Biol Sci Med Sci 56:M146–M156
2. Clegg A, Young J, Iliffe S et al (2013) Frailty in elderly people. Lancet 381:752–762
3. Rockwood K, Song X, Mitnitski A (2011) Changes in relative fitness and frailty across the adult lifespan: evidence from the Canadian National Population Health Survey. Can Med Assoc J 183:E487–E494
4. Mitnitski AB, Mogilner AJ, Rockwood K (2001) Accumulation of deficits as a proxy measure of aging. Sci World J 1:323–336
5. Mitnitski AB, Graham JE, Mogilner AJ et al (2002) Frailty, fitness and late-life mortality in relation to chronological and biological age. BMC Geriatr 2:1
6. Buta BJ, Walston JD, Godino JG et al (2016) Frailty assessment instruments: systematic characterization of the uses and contexts of highly-cited instruments. Ageing Res Rev 26:53–61
7. Theou O, Brothers TD, Mitnitski A et al (2013) Operationalization of frailty using eight commonly used scales and comparison of their ability to predict all-cause mortality. J Am Geriatr Soc 61:1537–1551
8. Morley JE, Malmstrom TK, Miller DK (2012) A simple frailty questionnaire (FRAIL) predicts outcomes in middle aged African Americans. J Nutr Health Aging 16:601–608
9. Cherubini A, Demougeot L, Jentoft AC et al (2015) Relationship between the Gérontopôle Frailty Screening Tool and the frailty phenotype in primary care. Eur Geriatr Med 6:518–522
10. Jones DM, Song X, Rockwood K (2004) Operationalizing a frailty index from a standardized comprehensive geriatric assessment. J Am Geriatr Soc 52:1929–1933
11. Cerreta F, Ankri J, Bowen D et al (2016) Baseline frailty evaluation in drug development. J Frailty Aging 5:139–140
12. Bruyère O, Buckinx F, Beaudart C et al (2017) How clinical practitioners assess frailty in their daily practice: an international survey. Aging Clin Exp Res 29:905–912
13. Collard RM, Boter H, Schoevers RA et al (2012) Prevalence of frailty in community-dwelling older persons: a systematic review. J Am Geriatr Soc 60:1487–1492
14. Santos-Eggimann B, Cuénoud P, Spagnoli J et al (2009) Prevalence of frailty in middle-aged and older community-dwelling Europeans living in 10 countries. J Gerontol A Biol Sci Med Sci 64:675–681
15. Bandeen-Roche K, Seplaki CL, Huang J et al (2015) Frailty in older adults: a nationally representative profile in the United States. J Gerontol A Biol Sci Med Sci 70:1427–1434
16. Mitnitski A, Song X, Rockwood K (2013) Assessing biological aging: the origin of deficit accumulation. Biogerontology 14:709–717
17. Gill TM, Gahbauer EA, Allore HG et al (2006) L. Transitions between frailty states among community-living older persons. Arch Intern Med 166:418–423
18. Espinoza SE, Jung I, Hazuda H (2012) Frailty transitions in the San Antonio longitudinal study of aging. J Am Geriatr Soc 60:652–660
19. Shardell M, D'Adamo C, Alley DE et al (2012) Serum 25-hydroxyvitamin D, transitions between frailty states, and mortality in older adults: the Invecchiare in Chianti Study. J Am Geriatr Soc 60:256–264
20. Lee JSW, Auyeung T-W, Leung J et al (2014) Transitions in frailty states among community-living older adults and their associated factors. J Am Med Dir Assoc 15:281–286

21. Pollack LR, Litwack-Harrison S, Cawthon PM et al (2017) Patterns and predictors of frailty transitions in older men: The osteoporotic fractures in men study. J Am Geriatr Soc 65(11):2473–2479
22. World Health Organization (2015) WHO, Geneva. http://www.who.int/ageing/publications/world-report-2015/en/. Accessed 10 Oct 2017
23. Cesari M, Prince M, Thiyagarajan JA et al (2016) Frailty: an emerging public health priority. J Am Med Dir Assoc 17:188–192
24. Fiatarone MA, O'Neill EF, Ryan ND et al (1994) Exercise training and nutritional supplementation for physical frailty in very elderly people. N Engl J Med 330:1769–1775
25. Gill TM, Baker DI, Gottschalk M et al (2002) A program to prevent functional decline in physically frail, elderly persons who live at home. N Engl J Med 347:1068–1074
26. Pahor M, Guralnik JM, Ambrosius WT et al (2014) Effect of structured physical activity on prevention of major mobility disability in older adults: the LIFE study randomized clinical trial. JAMA 311:2387–2396
27. Cesari M, Vellas B, Hsu F-C et al (2015) A physical activity intervention to treat the frailty syndrome in older persons—results from the LIFE-P study. J Gerontol A Biol Sci Med Sci 70:216–222
28. Theou O, Stathokostas L, Roland KP et al (2011) The effectiveness of exercise interventions for the management of frailty: a systematic review. J Aging Res 2011:569194
29. Puts MTE, Toubasi S, Andrew MK et al (2017) Interventions to prevent or reduce the level of frailty in community-dwelling older adults: a scoping review of the literature and international policies. Age Ageing 46:383–392
30. Frost R, Belk C, Jovicic A et al (2017) Health promotion interventions for community-dwelling older people with mild or pre-frailty: a systematic review and meta-analysis. BMC Geriatr 17:157
31. Ekdahl AW, Sjöstrand F, Ehrenberg A et al (2015) Frailty and comprehensive geriatric assessment organized as CGA-ward or CGA-consult for older adult patients in the acute care setting: a systematic review and meta-analysis. Eur Geriatr Med 6:523–540
32. De Almeida MJ, Hermans K, Audenhove CV et al (2015) Evaluations of home care interventions for frail older persons using the interRAI Home Care Instrument: a systematic review of the literature. J Am Med Dir Assoc 16:173.e1–173.10
33. Mor V, Intrator O, Fries BE et al (1997) Changes in hospitalization associated with introducing the Resident Assessment Instrument. J Am Geriatr Soc 45:1002–1010
34. Marzetti E, Calvani R, Tosato M et al (2017) Physical activity and exercise as countermeasures to physical frailty and sarcopenia. Aging Clin Exp Res 29:35–42
35. Landi F, Cesari M, Calvani R et al (2017) The "Sarcopenia and Physical fRailty IN older people: multi-componenT Treatment strategies" (SPRINTT) randomized controlled trial: design and methods. Aging Clin Exp Res 29:89–100

7 Cardiovascular, Cerebrovascular, and Renovascular Consequences of Ageing May Be Challenged

Timo E. Strandberg

Key Messages

- Although vascular disease is a frequent companion of ageing, it is not an inevitable process and cannot be considered a normal ageing phenomenon.
- The development with ageing of cardio-, cerebro-, and reno-vascular diseases can already be challenged through early and effective control of risk factors, by healthy lifestyle and drugs already available.
- Plasma low density lipoprotein (LDL) level is the main predisposing factor for atherosclerotic vascular disease, whereas hypertension, smoking, and hyperglycemia are precipitating factors for clinical events.
- Hypertension is considered the most important single risk factor of mortality and disability.
- Many geriatric syndromes may actually have vascular origins: macrovascular events (infarctions in coronary or cerebral arteries), microvascular disorders (small vessel disease) lead to white matter lesions in the brain, chronic kidney disease, and geriatric heart disease (heart failure, atrial fibrillation).
- In general, best results of risk factor treatments are achieved when started in midlife and continued to old age.

"You are as old as your arteries"

T. E. Strandberg
Helsinki University Central Hospital, Universities of Helsinki and Oulu, Helsinki, Finland
e-mail: timo.strandberg@oulu.fi

J.-P. Michel (ed.), *Prevention of Chronic Diseases and Age-Related Disability*, Practical Issues in Geriatrics, https://doi.org/10.1007/978-3-319-96529-1_7

7.1 Introduction

Although vascular disease is a frequent companion of ageing, it is not an inevitable process and cannot be considered a normal ageing phenomenon. This notion is supported by findings in primitive populations, like the Bolivian Amazon Tsimane people, who have both low levels of traditional risk factors, such as low density lipoprotein (LDL) cholesterol, and very low prevalence of coronary artery disease [1]. Moreover, were advanced atherosclerosis an unavoidable part of ageing, we should find it eventually in all individuals. This seems not to be the case, as there is postmortem evidence of a 115-year-old Dutch woman to be free of significant atherosclerosis [2]. The coronary "epidemic" of the twentieth-century and early vascular ageing (EVA, [3]) simply reflect longer life and a greater prevalence of risk factors such as dyslipidemia and hypertension. Common is not a synonym for normal.

Although progress in vascular research will undoubtedly produce more and more sophisticated methods to preserve vascular function and health, the development of cardio-, cerebro-, and reno-vascular diseases can already be challenged through early and effective control of risk factors (aggressive decrease of atherosclerosis modifiers, ADAM, [3]) by lifestyle and drugs already available. But results are the better, the earlier prevention is begun (Fig. 7.1).

7.2 Pathophysiology

In the vessel wall, macro- and microvascular dysfunction is the primary phenomenon in the pathophysiology of vascular disease (Fig. 7.2). Upstream factors include oxidative stress, shear and wall stress, and inflammation [4–6] which in turn are caused by various risk factors, especially hypertension, dyslipidemia, obesity, and hyperglycemia. Factors related to ageing—senescence and growth arrest—contribute and

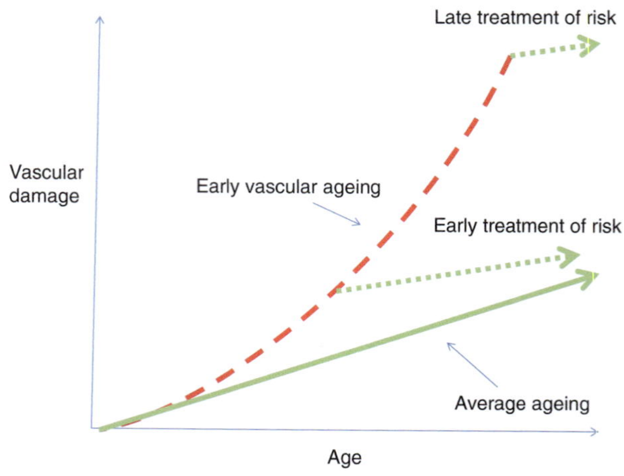

Fig. 7.1 Time scheme to challenge early vascular ageing and development of vascular disease by risk factor treatment (modified from [3])

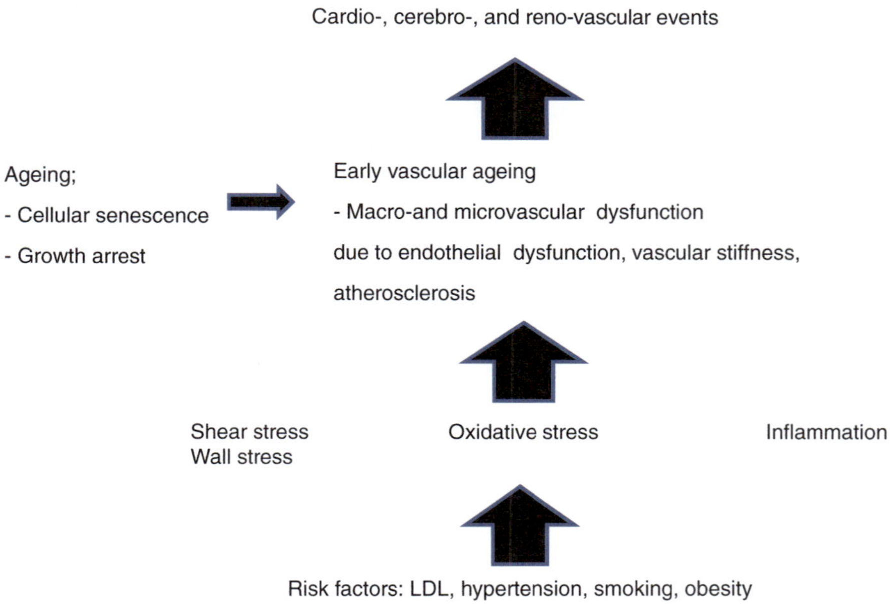

Fig. 7.2 Mechanisms of vascular damage leading clinical events

amplify pathologic process. Subclinical target organ damage in the vessel wall (intima-media thickness, stiffness, endothelial dysfunction), heart (left ventricle hypertrophy), and kidney (microalbuminuria) can be measured to assess the development of vascular damage before clinical events like myocardial infarction, stroke, heart, or kidney failure occur.

7.3 Ageing and Risk Factors

Chronological age plays a dual role in the context of cardiovascular risk factors and diseases. On the one hand, ageing-related changes in the organism (cellular senescence, growth arrest) predispose to pathological factors; on the other hand, age of an individual simply reflects the time of predisposition to the total burden of risk factors. Consequently, chronological age is a major risk factor for any chronic disease, but this association may disappear, if analyses are adjusted for markers of biological age, such as frailty, and risk factors.

Traditional risk factors consist of predisposing and precipitating risk factors. Several lines of evidence show that plasma low density lipoprotein (LDL) level is the main predisposing factor for atherosclerotic vascular disease [7, 8], whereas hypertension, smoking, and hyperglycemia are precipitating factors for clinical events. If LDL cholesterol level is chronically very low (0.5–1.0 mmol/L) as in some vegetarian cultures or in persons with mutations leading to low plasma LDL cholesterol levels (loss of function of pro-protein convertase subtilisin/kexin type 9

[PCSK9] gene, [6]), atherosclerotic cardiovascular disease does not develop or develops very slowly despite other risk factors. An extreme case is the loss of apoprotein B (ApoB), main component of LDL, which has been associated with longevity and remarkably clean arteries [9].

However, when LDL cholesterol levels are at typical “Western” levels (1.8 mmol/L and usually much higher), other risk factors act as precipitators and therefore individuals with several concomitant risk factors (high-risk individuals) tend to have clinical events earlier.

The effects of risk factors may be resisted by individual protective factors, which are often poorly understood. These can be environmental, healthy lifestyle-related, or genetic. Protective factors help to explain, why few individuals live a long life despite regular smoking or unhealthy diet. Homeostatic mechanisms (low cholesterol absorption/high excretion) can keep plasma LDL cholesterol levels low despite unhealthy diet. Consequences of high blood pressure may be less effectively protected from increased wall and shear stress over the years, and it is no wonder that hypertension is considered the most important single risk factor of mortality and disability [10].

7.4 Cardio-, Cerebro- and Reno-Vascular Diseases and Their Life-Course Development

Among people ≥60 years, it is currently estimated that 30.3%, 15.1%, 9.5%, 7.5% and 6.6% of the disease burden is due to cardiovascular disease, cancer, chronic respiratory disease, musculoskeletal disease, and neurological and mental disorders, respectively [11, 12]. Importantly, it is considered that even 2/3 of top 15 causes of death are lifestyle related, potentially preventable, or at least possible to postpone. This especially applies to atherosclerotic vascular disease, but in order to attain best results, prevention should start early. Non-communicable diseases have a long time of development, for example, first signs of atherosclerosis (intima-media thickening, fatty streaks) can be discerned already in youth [13] although clinical events (infarctions, stroke) occur in midlife or later. Sadly, effective treatment is often postponed and especially evidence-based drug treatments, such as statins and anti-hypertensives, are initiated relatively late in the pathological process and therapeutic effects are less optimal or may be even null. In risk factor control, the importance is “not only **how much**, but **how long”** (Fig. 7.1).

Fortunately, better control of hypercholesterolemia, hypertension and smoking at the population level and through lifestyle changes during the last decades has led to dramatic drop in coronary heart disease and stroke among people <65 years of age in many countries, for example in Finland where in the 1960s men used to lead world statistics in coronary deaths [14]. A positive consequence of this development has been that people enter old age in better health, and are living longer.

A crucial question is, however, will the extra years be spent with sustained quality of life and functionality? Various possibilities exist. The ideal scenario would be the “compression of morbidity”, a vision introduced by Fries in 1980: time of disease and disability would be compressed to a short period just before death [15]; the worst scenario in turn that most of extra years is spent with disability and comorbidity, in other words, healthy lifespan is not prolonged ("expansion of morbidity"). It is currently obscure which scenario will prevail and probably there are also differences between societies and population groups [12].

Another characteristic of the current development is that in old age diseases may manifest in different forms, further complicated and modified by the ageing process. In addition to macrovascular events (infarctions in coronary or cerebral arteries), microvascular disorders (small vessel disease) lead to white matter lesions in the brain, chronic kidney disease and geriatric heart disease (heart failure, atrial fibrillation).

Prolongation of lifespan also increases risk for multimorbidity which complicates treatments and leads to polypharmacy with problems of its own. Multimorbidity is also closely intertwined with various geriatric syndromes [16], such as frailty, which should be considered as important clinical endpoints of midlife risk factors.

7.5 Vascular Ageing Is Also Related to Geriatric Syndromes

Geriatric syndromes predispose older people to disability and death [16]. They are common among older people, and often coexist with other diseases, especially cardiovascular diseases and diabetes; many geriatric syndromes may actually have vascular origins [17]. Core pathophysiologic disorders include atherosclerosis, arterial stiffening, small vessel disease and amyloid angiopathy. They act in concert to induce infarction and hemorrhage in larger and smaller vessels, in the brain they predispose to white matter lesions and blood-brain barrier dysfunction, which in turn are related to cognitive decline, depression, and delirium. Vascular origins may offer good possibilities for long-term prevention.

7.6 Midlife Risk Factors for Cardiovascular Diseases and Geriatric Syndromes

In the following the focus will be on the most prevalent cardiovascular diseases of older people [11, 12]. Except frailty, cognitive disorders, geriatric heart disease, research is so far limited for midlife origins of geriatric syndromes.

7.6.1 Coronary Heart Disease

The most important predisposing and long-term risk factor is dyslipidemia, especially high LDL cholesterol level. LDL is a sine qua non for atherosclerotic plaques [7], and inflammation enters secondarily. On the other hand, precipitating risk factors (hypertension, smoking, diabetes) are associated with the probability of clinical events in short term (5–10 years).

7.6.2 Cerebrovascular Diseases, "Stroke"

Long-term hypertension is the most important risk factor for both ischemic and hemorrhagic stroke [10], whereas chronic or paroxysmal atrial fibrillation is usually associated with embolic stroke. Obesity contributes to ischemic and hemorrhagic stroke, and although hypercholesterolemia has not consistently predicted stroke, cholesterol lowering with statins has been shown to decrease also ischemic stroke [7].

7.6.3 Chronic Kidney Disease

Hypertension is the most important midlife risk factor accompanied by obesity and hyperglycemia [10]. Chronic kidney disease is also associated with increased cardiovascular disease risk.

7.6.4 Hypertensive Heart Disease

Hypertension is also an important risk factor for heart failure [10], especially the form with reduced ejection fraction (HFrEF). However, because coronary heart disease is an important cause of HFrEF, hypercholesterolemia is also indirectly involved.

7.6.5 Atrial Fibrillation

This arrhythmia is usually associated with other heart disease (coronary heart disease, heart failure) with their general risk factors. AF predisposes to atrial thrombosis and cardiac emboli leading to cerebrovascular occlusion and stroke [18].

7.6.6 Frailty and Sarcopenia

If frailty is defined as an index consisting of diseases and disabilities [19], it is natural that their risk factors are associated with frailty. There is also some data about long-term risk factors of frailty defined as a phenotype. Observational data suggest that physical inactivity and obesity in midlife are independent predictors of physical frailty [19, 20]. Also total cardiovascular disease risk in midlife predispose to frailty in old age [20]. Inflammation and other emerging risk factors are associated with frailty and sarcopenia, but these may be more downstream factors, and no long-term studies are available specifically about the inflammatory state in midlife.

7.7 Levels of Prevention

The majority of cardio- cerebro-, and reno-vascular events are caused by "traditional" risk factors that can be controlled or modified. These include hypertension, dyslipidemia (hypercholesterolemia), overweight/obesity, smoking, and physical inactivity. Depending on age and target population, different levels of prevention may be distinguished:

7.7.1 Primordial Prevention

This aims to prevent development of traditional risk factors [21]. Genetic and ageing-related factors cannot (as yet) be manipulated, but emerging therapies may mimic actions of mutations and longevity mechanisms. Examples include synthesis inhibition of PCSK9 protein leading to very low levels to LDL [7]. Currently it is possible to promote primordial prevention via lifestyle (not smoking, low sodium diet to prevent hypertension, vegetarian diet to prevent dyslipidemia, physical activity and weight control to prevent obesity etc.), but this must be done early in life and also at the societal level through legislation [22].

7.7.2 Primary Prevention

This implies modifying adverse levels of risk factors before they cause clinical disease. This can be attained with intensive lifestyle modifications, but because processes have usually been long-standing combining drug treatment with lifestyle modifications is more effective.

7.7.3 Secondary Prevention

This is similar to primary prevention but is started after a clinical event in order to prevent recurrent events. Evidence-based drug treatment, such as statins, is usually indicated.

7.8 Treatment of Risk Factors in Different Phases of Life Course

In observational studies the relationship between risk factors and disease often reverses during the life course, but it is very important to discern endogenous (due to clinical or subclinical disease, frailty) and exogenous (due to lifestyle or drug treatment) risk factor change. For example, high blood pressure, high cholesterol and high body mass index clearly predict mortality when measured in midlife, whereas there is necessarily no association, or even reverse ("obesity paradox") when the risk factor is measured in old age. Several factors may explain these discrepancies. It is possible that individuals surviving to old age have protective factors, or risk factors may change due to diseases and frailty, which are the true explanations for poorer prognosis. Moreover, cross-sectional measurement of risk factors in old age does not necessarily reflect the risk factor burden earlier in life. Also medications among older people alter risk factor status. On the other hand, the effect of risk factors may be age-dependent, although evidences from randomized controlled trials do not generally support this notion. Antihypertensive drugs prevent clinical events even when started in patients aged 80 years or older, cholesterol lowering with statins has reduced cardiovascular events at least up to 80 years. There is not much research about treatment of obesity in old age, but there is no reason to doubt that calorie reduction combined with physical activity would not as such be beneficial, if development of sarcopenia or nutritional deficiencies is avoided.

Because chronic diseases, such as cardiovascular diseases, take decades to develop, treatment of risk factors started in old age or in terminal stage (heart or kidney failure, dementia) is often "too little, too late".

7.8.1 Midlife

In general, best results of risk factor treatments are achieved when started in midlife and continued to old age. Table 7.1 presents midlife characteristics which are associated with healthy ageing [23]. There is increasing evidence that they would also be associated with reduced risk of geriatric syndromes, such as frailty and dementia in old age.

These protective factors should be promoted at various levels, both at societal level (anti-smoking laws, physical activity-friendly environment, reduction of salt or added sugar in foods), and at individual level through lifestyle and drug treatment as needed. Especially antihypertensive drugs, statins, aspirin, and tobacco cessation drugs are evidence-based therapies to decrease cardiovascular risk and common clinical events with minor adverse effects [24]. However, it is more difficult to demonstrate benefits with a controlled trial in the prevention of geriatric syndromes like dementia [25], because duration should probably be more than the usual 2–5 years.

Table 7.1 Midlife characteristics which are associated with healthy ageing (modified from "Life's simple 7", [23])

• No smoking
• "Vascular healthy" diet
• Physical activity at least 30 min daily
• Body mass index below 25 kg/m^2, no "abdominal obesity"
• Blood pressure below 120/80 mmHg
• Low density lipoprotein (LDL) cholesterol below 3 mmol/L
• No diabetes

A highly interesting idea to improve adherence and prevent clinical events is the polypill concept [26], a combination of low doses of cheap antihypertensive and statin drugs for individuals above 55 years. The benefits are getting supportive evidence from clinical studies and if preventing or postponing vascular disease would also prevent geriatric syndromes, a polypill would be an easy and cost-effective solution to promote healthy ageing.

7.8.2 Old Age

In general there are no age limits for continuing preventive measures started earlier life. The decision to discontinue ("deprescribe") a medication is dependent on assessment of risk-benefit. In terminal stage, treatments are naturally directed away from prevention towards palliation. Lifestyle modifications are challenging in old age, although stopping smoking, eating a heart and brain healthy diet, and physical activity are considered useful at any age. Starting preventive medications, such as statins or anti-hypertensives, in people older than 80 years needs individual decisions [27, 28] and are more important in secondary prevention. In the case of atrial fibrillation, anticoagulation with warfarin or direct anticoagulants is an effective form of therapy to prevent cerebrovascular disease also in old age [29].

Conclusions

In the prevention of cardio-, cerebro-, and reno-vascular diseases, it is important to recognize the long-term development of these conditions. In ageing societies they constitute an enormous burden for health and nursing care. It is also important to realize that excellent possibilities already exist to prevent these conditions and promote healthy ageing, but for best results prevention should start early in persons at risk.

References

1. Kaplan H, Thompson RC, Trumble BC et al (2017) Coronary atherosclerosis in indigenous south American Tsimane: a cross-sectional cohort study. Lancet 389:1730–1739
2. Den Dunnen WF, Brouwer WH, Bijlard E et al (2008) No disease in the brain of a 115-year-old woman. Neurobiol Aging 29:1127–1132
3. Nilsson PM, Boutouyrie P, Laurent S (2009) Vascular aging. A tale of EVA and ADAM in cardiovascular risk assessment and prevention. Hypertension 54:3–10
4. Green DJ, Hopman MTE, Padilla J et al (2017) Vascular adaptation to exercise in humans: role of hemodynamic stimuli. Physiol Rev 97:495–528
5. Guzik TJ, Touyz RM (2017) Oxidative stress, inflammation, and vascular aging in hypertension. Hypertension 70:660–667
6. Seals DR, Kaplon RE, Gioscia RA, LaRocca TJ (2014) You're only as old as your arteries: translational strategies for preserving vascular endothelial function with aging. Physiology 29:250–264
7. Goldstein JL, Brown MS (2015) A century of cholesterol and coronaries: from plaques to genes to statins. Cell 161:161–172

8. Ference BA, Ginsberg HN, Graham I et al (2017) Low-density lipoproteins cause atherosclerotic cardiovascular disease. 1. Evidence from genetic, epidemiologic, and clinical studies. A consensus statement from the European Atherosclerosis Society Consensus Panel. Eur Heart J 38(32):2459–2472. https://doi.org/10.1093/eurheartj/ehx144 [Epub ahead of print]
9. Kahn JA, Glueck CJ (1978) Familial hypobetalipoproteinemia. Absence of atherosclerosis in a postmortem study. JAMA 240:47–48
10. Poulter NR, Probhakaran D, Caulfield M (2015) Hypertension. Lancet 386:801–812
11. WHO (2015) World report on ageing and health. WHO, Geneva
12. Prince MJ, Guo Y, Gutierrez Robledo LM et al (2015) The burden of disease in older people and implications for health policy and practice. Lancet 385:549–546
13. Raitakari OT, Juonala M, Kähönen M et al (2003) Cardiovascular risk factors in childhood and carotid artery intima-media thickness in adulthood: the cardiovascular risk in young Finns study. JAMA 290:2277–2283
14. Jousilahti P, Laatikainen T, Peltonen M et al (2016) Primary prevention and risk factor reduction in coronary heart disease mortality among working aged men and women in eastern Finland over 40 years: population based observational study. BMJ 352:i721. https://doi.org/10.1136/bmj.i721
15. Fries JF (1980) Aging, natural death, and the compression of morbidity. N Engl J Med 303:130–135
16. Inouye SK, Studenski S, Tinetti ME, Kuchel GA (2007) Geriatric syndromes: clinical, research, and policy implications of a core geriatric concept. J Am Geriatr Soc 55:780–791
17. Strandberg TE, Pitkälä KH, Tilvis RS et al (2013) Geriatric syndromes—vascular disorders? Ann Med 45:265–273
18. Paulus Kirchhof P, Benussi S, Kotecha D (2016) 2016 ESC guidelines for the management of atrial fibrillation developed in collaboration with EACTS. Eur Heart J 37:2893–2962
19. Strandberg TE, Pitkälä K, Tilvis RS (2011) Frailty in older people. Eur Geriatr Med 2:344–355
20. Strandberg TE, Sirola J, Pitkälä KH et al (2012) Association of midlife obesity and cardiovascular risk with old age frailty: a 26-year follow-up of initially healthy men. Int J Obes 36:1153–1157
21. Weintraub WS, Daniels SR, Burke LE et al (2011) Value of primordial and primary prevention for cardiovascular disease. A policy statement of the American Heart Association. Circulation 124:967–990
22. US Preventive Services Task Force (2017) Behavioral counseling to promote a healthful diet and physical exercise for cardiovascular disease prevention in adults without cardiovascular risk factors. JAMA 318:167–174
23. Lloyd-Jones DM, Hong Y, Labarthe D et al (2010) Defining and setting national goals for cardiovascular health promotion and disease reduction: the American Heart Association's strategic impact goal through 2020 and beyond. Circulation 121:586–613
24. Karmali KN, Lloyd-Jones DM, Berendsen MA et al (2016) Drugs for primary prevention of atherosclerotic cardiovascular disease. An overview of systematic reviews. JAMA Cardiol 1:341–349
25. Andrieu S, Coley N, Lovestone S et al (2015) Prevention of sporadic Alzheimer's disease: lessons learned from clinical trials and future directions. Lancet 14:926
26. Bramlage P, Sims H, Minguet J, Ferrero C (2017) The polypill: an effective approach to increasing adherence and reducing cardiovascular event risk. Eur J Prev Cardiol 24(3):297–310
27. Strandberg TE, Kolehmainen L, Vuorio A (2014) Evaluation and treatment of older patients with hypercholesterolemia. JAMA 312:1136–1144
28. Benetos A, Rossignol P, Cherubini A et al (2015) Polypharmacy in the aging patient: management of hypertension in octogenarians. JAMA 314:170–180
29. Wehling M, Collins R, Gil VM et al (2017) Appropriateness of oral anticoagulants for the long-term treatment of atrial fibrillation in older people. Drugs Aging 34:499–507

The New Ways of Preventing and Treating Diabetes Mellitus

8

Peter Fasching

Abbreviations

BMI	Body mass index
CV	Cardiovascular
CVD	Cardiovascular disease
CVOT	Cardiovascular outcome trial
DPP	Diabetes Prevention Program [14]
DPP-4-I	Dipeptidyl-peptidase 4 inhibitors
DPPOS	Diabetes Prevention Program Outcome Study [15]
DPS	Diabetes Prevention Study [13]
GLP1-RA	Glucagon-like-peptide 1 receptor agonist
HbA1c	Glycosylated hemoglobin A1c
HR	Hazard ratio
IDF	International Diabetes Federation
sGLT2-I	Sodium-glucose-transporter 2 inhibitors
SSB	Sugar-sweetened beverages
T1D	Diabetes mellitus type 1
T2D	Diabetes mellitus type 2

P. Fasching
5th Internal Department with Endocrinology, Rheumatology and Acute Geriatrics, Wilhelminenspital of the City of Vienna, Vienna, Austria
e-mail: peter.fasching@wienkav.at

J.-P. Michel (ed.), *Prevention of Chronic Diseases and Age-Related Disability*, Practical Issues in Geriatrics, https://doi.org/10.1007/978-3-319-96529-1_8

Key Messages

- According to the Diabetes Atlas 2017, it is estimated that worldwide, 425 million aged 20–79 years are suffering from both diagnosed and undiagnosed diabetes.
- Over 60% of adults aged over 65 years have 2 or more chronic conditions. Socioeconomically disadvantaged individuals have a higher burden of multimorbidity.
- For all people, testing for dysglycemia should begin at the age of 45 years. Testing HbA1c alone is neither sensitive nor specific enough for detecting pre-diabetes in big cohorts. Fasting glucose on the other hand is specific but not very sensitive. Thus, broad population-based "screen and treat" policies alone are unlikely to have substantial impact on the worsening epidemic of T2D.
- In general, prevention of overweight and obesity in adolescence and midlife is one of the most important determinants of preventing development of diabetes in further life.
- Lifestyle interventions appear more sustainable to prevent diabetes in comparison to pharmaceutical approaches which loose efficacy after stopping and bear the risk of side-effects.
- If T2D is present, besides adequate lifestyle modification modern pharmaceutical strategies are required to safely control hyperglycemia in order to prevent severe acute and chronic complications, especially severe hypoglycemia and premature kidney and eye disease, cardiovascular complications, and death.

8.1 Introduction

The number of patients with T2D mellitus (T2D) is steeply increasing. According to the Diabetes Atlas 2017 published yearly by the International Diabetes Federation (IDF), it is estimated for all forms of both diagnosed and undiagnosed diabetes that worldwide 425 million aged 20–79 years are affected, a number which will rise to 629 million people in 2045. Nowadays 1 in 2 patients is undiagnosed, two third of diabetic patients are in working age between 20 and 64 years [1].

In Germany, age- and sex-standardized all-cause mortality is almost twice as high for adults with T2D as for adults without T2D. T2D's associated excess risk for mortality appears to be most pronounced in younger adults and among those unaware of their disease [2].

In the USA in 2010, over 60% of adults aged 65 years or more had two or more chronic conditions as did a third of adults aged 45–64 years. Socioeconomically disadvantaged individuals have a higher burden of multimorbidity, and they develop multiple chronic conditions 10–15 years earlier than those who are more socioeconomically advantaged. People with multimorbidity are common users of health care, generate costs, and are at increased risk for adverse events. Most of these individuals are cared for practitioners with inadequate expertise in geriatrics or multimorbidity [3].

Thus, strategies in midlife to prevent development of diabetes mellitus, mostly T2D, and its negative late sequela for health are of imminent importance for the individual as well as for societies and health systems [4]. If diabetes is diagnosed, adequate lifestyle modification and modern pharmaceutical strategies are required to safely control hyperglycemia in order to prevent severe acute and chronic complications [5].

In this context, management of body weight seems to play a crucial role in prevention and also treatment of diabetes mellitus and its further prognosis.

8.2 Body Weight Management, Risk of T2D, and Mortality

In general, prevention of overweight and obesity in adolescence and midlife is one of the most important determinants of preventing development of diabetes in further life. According to a large population-based study, weight maintenance in adulthood is strongly associated with reduced incident diabetes risk, and there is considerable potential for diabetes prevention in promoting this as a whole population strategy [6].

Following the results of the Global BMI Mortality Collaboration in non-diabetic populations, the association of both overweight and obesity with higher all-cause mortality is broadly consistent in different continents. For BMI over 25.0 kg/m^2, the Hazard Ratio (HR) for increased mortality per 5 kg/m^2 units higher BMI was 1.39 in Europe and 1.29 in North America. This HR was greater in younger than in older people (1.52 for BMI measured at 35–49 years vs. 1.21 for BMI measured at 70–89 years, $p < 0.0001$) [7].

On the other hand, in patients with already existing T2D an "obesity paradoxon" appears concerning the risk of mortality, also modified by age. This means that older diabetic persons have a better prognosis when they are overweight: A recent meta-analysis including 250,016 patients shows a significantly lower risk of all-cause mortality in overweight patients with diabetes compared with normal patients. However, the survival benefits were only observed among the elderly patients older than 65 years of life. Furthermore, the beneficial prognostic impacts of overweight and obesity were attenuated with clinical follow-up duration [8].

When differentiating individuals according to their state of glycemia by group in a recently published cohort study optimal BMI (kg/m^2) for the lowest mortality by group was 23.5–27.9 (normoglycemia), 25–27.9 (impaired fasting glucose), 25–29.4 (newly diagnosed diabetes), and 26.5–29.4 (prevalent diabetes). The relationship between worsening diabetes status and higher mortality was stronger with lower BMI, especially at younger ages. Given the same BMI, people with prevalent diabetes had higher mortality compared with those with newly diagnosed diabetes, and this was more striking in women than in men. *U*-curve relationships existed regardless of diabetes status. Optimal BMI for lowest mortality became gradually higher with worsening diabetes for each gender and age group [9].

8.3 Screening for T2D in Midlife

For all people, testing for dysglycemia should begin at the age of 45 years. If tests are normal, repeat testing carried out at 3-year interval is reasonable. To test for T2D or pre-diabetes, fasting plasma glucose, 2-h plasma glucose during 75-g oral glucose tolerance test, and glycosylated hemoglobin 1c (HbA1c) are equally appropriate [10]. According to a recent meta-analysis however, HbA1c is neither sensitive nor specific for detecting pre-diabetes in big cohorts. On the other hand, fasting glucose is specific but not sensitive. Yet, on the basis of this systematic review, interventions in people classified through screening as having pre-diabetes have some efficacy in preventing or delaying onset of T2D in specific trial populations. In contrary, in clinical practice as routine screening methodology per se is inaccurate, many people will receive an incorrect diagnosis and be referred to interventions while others will be falsely reassured and not offered the intervention. These findings from the review suggest that "screen and treat" policies alone are unlikely to have substantial impact on the worsening epidemic of T2D [11].

8.4 Strategies for Prevention in High Risk Populations and/or Reversal of Manifest T2D

Weight reduction of 15 kg or more in individuals aged 20–65 years with a body mass index (BMI) of 27–45 kg/m^2 and a known duration of non-insulin requiring diabetes of less than 6 years leads to a complete diabetes remission of 86% of included patients in an open-label trial in primary care. Overall, the study results show that, after 12 months of nutritional intervention, almost half of the participants in the active study arm achieved remission to a non-diabetic state and was off anti-diabetic drugs. Thus, remission of T2D appears as realistic target also for primary care although sustainability of this effect has to be proven over a longer period of time [12].

From a pathophysiological point of view, weight loss results in improved insulin sensitivity in muscles and liver, decreases intra-organ fat content, and might improve insulin secretion. In the long term, weight loss might help to preserve ß-cell mass, maybe by decreased fat content of the pancreas. The role of physical activity and quality of diet, such as dietary fiber and fatty acid composition should not be forgotten when considering the long-term success of prevention and treatment of T2D [12].

Lifestyle interventions in middle-aged pre-diabetic cohorts with 7% weight loss in the first 6 months of intervention and a goal for physical activity of at least 150 min of moderate-intensity physical activity per week similar in intensity to brisk walking reduced the incidence of overt T2D by 58% over about 3 years of observation versus control in the Finish Diabetes Prevention Study (DPS) as well as in the American Diabetes Prevention Program (DPP) [13, 14].

Long-term follow-ups of these two studies have shown sustained reduction in the rate of conversion to T2D: 43% reduction at 7 years in the Diabetes Prevention

Study (DPS), and 34% reduction at 10 years and 27% reduction at 15 years in the Diabetes Prevention Program Outcomes Study (DPPOS), an observational extension of the DPP [4].

As to pharmaceutical attempts of T2D prevention, in the DPP metformin reduced the incidence of new diabetes by 31% compared with placebo after an average follow-up of 2.8 years, with a greater effect in those who were more obese, younger, had a higher fasting glucose or a history of gestational diabetes. DPPOS addressed the longer term effects of metformin, showing a risk reduction of 18% over 10 and 15 years post-randomization. Metformin treatment for diabetes prevention was estimated to be cost-saving. In the DPP, obese participants with BMI >35 kg/m^2 were more responsive to metformin than placebo, with a 53% risk reduction for diabetes but only a 3% reduction in those with BMI 22 to <30 kg/m^2. Although not significant, metformin appeared more effective in younger participants compared with placebo, reducing diabetes onset by 44% in those 24–44 years old vs. 11% in those >60 years of age at study entry [15].

Nonetheless, metformin is not licensed for prevention of T2D, nor is any other pharmaceutical compound licensed for that indication for the time being, although in pre-diabetic cohorts the thiazolidinediones (glitazones = insulin-sensitizers), rosiglitazone and pioglitazone, the alpha-glucosidase inhibitor acarbose, and the long-acting insulin analogon glargine could show reduction of new-onset diabetes in specific clinical trials [4]. The potential clinical role of Glucagon-Like-Peptide-1 receptor agonists (GLP-1-RA) like the subcutaneously injectable liraglutide for that purpose is still under investigation [16]. According to a recent meta-analysis, lifestyle interventions in general appear more sustainable concerning their preventive potential to prevent diabetes in comparison to different pharmaceutical approaches which—up to now—loose efficacy after stopping and wash out and bear the risk of side-effects (e.g., increased risk of bone fractures in postmenopausal women under glitazone treatment) [17].

8.5 Anti-Hypoglycemic Agents and Their Potential "Anti-Aging" Effects

In a recent meta-analysis, based on the findings of an observed reduction in all-cause mortality and diseases of aging independent on its effect on diabetes control, the hypothesis was put forward that metformin could be extending life and health spans by acting as geroprotective agent [18]. Although metformin's effect on clinical aging outcomes may still be considered speculative, the findings from studies into cellular and animal models and from observational and pilot human studies support the existence of beneficial effects on aging. At present, randomized clinical trials to evaluate metformin's clinical impact are ongoing [19].

In long-term clinical use however, it has to be borne in mind that metformin may lower vitamin B12 concentrations in blood consequently to impaired vitamin B12-absorption, as shown in the DPPOS [20]. This observation and consequently vitamin B12 supplementation, when necessary, seem important because an association exists between vitamin B12 deficit and development of geriatric syndromes, not determined if causal or not [21].

On the other hand, concerning incidence of Parkinson's disease, according to data from the Norwegian Prescription Database glitazone use was associated with a significantly lower incidence of Parkinson's disease compared with metformin-only use (hazard ratio, 0.72; confidence interval, 0.55–0.94; $p = 0.01$) during a 10-year observation period [22]. Further studies are warranted to confirm and understand the role of glitazones in neurodegeneration.

Also, the once-weekly GLP-1-RA exenatide LAR had positive effects on practically defined off-medication motor scores in non-diabetic patients with moderate Parkinson's disease, which were sustained beyond the period of exposure. Whether exenatide affects the underlying disease pathophysiology or simply induces long-lasting symptomatic effects on everyday symptoms remain uncertain and should be examined in longer trials [23].

8.6 Glycemic Control and Weight Management in Manifest Diabetes

For patients with both T1D and T2D mellitus, there are positive and statistically significant associations between being overweight or obese and having sub-optimal glycemic control [24].

In a meta-analysis at group level, weight loss in obese and overweight T2D patients is consistently accompanied by HbA1c reduction in a dose-dependent manner, corresponding to a mean HbA1c reduction of 0.1% per each kilogram of mean weight loss whereby HbA1c lowering is greater in populations with poor glycemic control than in well-controlled populations with the same degree of weight loss [25].

In an open-label study, 5-year outcome data showed that, among patients with T2D and a BMI of 27–43 kg/m^2, bariatric surgery plus intensive medical therapy was more effective than intensive medical therapy alone in decreasing, or in some cases resolving, hyperglycemia [26].

8.7 Nutrition, Diabetes Mellitus, and Successful Aging or Frailty

In the context of medically induced weight reduction, it has to be stated that to my knowledge no convincing studies are published which prove the long-term benefits on age-related disabilities, geriatric syndromes and/or mortality in obese persons over 65 years or older.

Yet, there is evidence that diet quality in later life may influence the development of frailty. Adherence to the Mediterranean diet seems to be particularly protective against developing frailty. This effect appears to be related predominantly to a higher intake in polyphenols. Overall, it seems that anorexia of aging and associated weight loss represents an important role in the pathophysiology of frailty [27].

Frailty is a common finding and may be present in 32–48% of adults aged 65 years and over with manifest T2D and is associated with adverse outcomes and reduced survival. Frailty is regarded as a pre-disability condition that creates opportunity for intervention to enhance functional performance [28] (see Chap. 7).

Thus, advice for iatrogenic weight reduction and management in older age must be given with caution and should be combined with an adequate supply of protein, vitamins and trace elements, and an exercise program to prevent myopenia.

The importance of understanding different levels of patient enthusiasm and different responses to exercise should guide the participatory phase of sarcopenic treatment [29].

Concerning intake of alcohol, in a large survey consumption of alcohol over 3–4 days per week is associated with the lowest risk of diabetes, even taking average weekly consumption into account. Compared with current alcohol consumers consuming <1 day/week, consumption of alcohol on 3–4 days weekly was associated with significantly lower risk for diabetes in men (HR 0.73) and women (HR 0.68) after adjusting for confounders and average weekly alcohol amount [30].

8.8 Diabetes Mellitus and Cardiovascular Disease (CVD)

For patients with T2D, cardiovascular disease (CVD) is the single most common cause of mortality. The average life expectancy of a 60-year-old male with T2D and no risk of cardiovascular (CV) disease (CVD) is 12 years less than his counterpart without diabetes, mostly owing to a 58% increase in risk in CV death [31].

Since autumn 2015 several published clinical cardiovascular outcomes trials (CVOTs) with new pharmaceutical compounds in the field of T2D have changed the knowledge how to select and prioritize glycemic treatment [5].

To date, in summer of 2018, empagliflozin and canagliflozin, two inhibitors of the sodium-glucose-transporter-2 system (sGLT-2-inhibitors) in the kidney, and liraglutide and semaglutide, two long-acting GLP-1 receptor agonists have proven to significantly reduce primary composite CV endpoints in T2D patients (partly empagliflozin and liraglutide also isolated CV and total mortality), mainly in those with pre-existing cardiovascular and/or multiple cardiovascular risk factors. Also secondary kidney endpoints were significantly reduced, clinically more relevant under sGLT-2 inhibition with empagliflozin and canagliflozin [5].

The short-acting GLP-RA lixisenatide and the long-acting GLP-1-RA exenatide LAR failed to show significant reduction in the composite primary endpoint, maybe due to different study designs and study populations [5].

More of those studies are to follow in the next years with similar compounds (i.e. dagliflozin and dulaglutide).

Several published CVOTs with oral dipeptidyp-peptidase-4 (DPP-4)-inhibitors (Alo-, Saxa-, Lina- and Sitagliptin) brought neutral results in cardiovascular outcomes versus placebo on top of standard diabetes therapy [5]. The patients at inclusion into those CVOTs were uniformly in the early 60s with about 60% of male predominance.

In light of these recent CVOTs in the field of diabetes mellitus, the diagnosis, assessment, treatment choice, and monitoring of patients with T2D and established CVD and/or chronic kidney disease (CKD) have to be considered in choice of anti-glycemic drugs together with existing guidelines [32].

Nonetheless, up to 2018, metformin stays the primary and basal therapeutic option, if not tolerated or contraindicated [5].

In contrast to insulin therapy and therapy with sulfonylurea or glinides, all the other and especially the modern therapeutic options have in common that they do not induce hypoglycemia per se (that means if not combined with insulin and sulfonylurea/glinides).

That seems of special importance because looking at routine data from over 300,000 people in the UK, collected between 2004 and 2015, it was found that lower levels of glycated hemoglobin—typically regarded as being good diabetes control—were associated with increased mortality risk, compared to moderate levels, especially in conjunction with intensive treatments that could cause hypoglycemia. Furthermore, the pattern of mortality in relation to glucose control differed in relation to differing types of diabetes drugs. Of most concern was an increase in mortality risk in those with low glycated hemoglobin reflecting "good control" with T2D who were treated with insulin and other glucose lowering drugs that induce hypoglycemia. In contrary, high levels of HbA1c were associated with the expected elevated mortality risk in regimes with low hypoglycemia risk [33]. Yet, it has to be stated that this association is observational and there is no scientific proof for causality.

As to statin intake and diabetes risk, a large meta-analysis comes to the conclusion that statin therapy is associated with an on average 9% increased risk for incident diabetes which was highest in trials with older participants. Clinical practice of obligatory statin use in patients with moderate or high CV risk or existing CVD should not change because this risk is low in absolute terms and especially negotiable when compared with the proven statin-induced reduction in CV events [34]. In a recent study, risk for new-onset diabetes in elderly women increased with increasing dose of statin from the hazard ratio of 1.17 for the lowest dose to 1.51 for the highest dose of statin. Overall, this equates to a number needed to harm (NNH) of 131 for 5 years of exposure to statins [35].

8.9 Public Health Considerations (Advice for Political Decision-Makers)

According to a recent study, functional impairment and decline are common in middle age, as are transitions from impairment to independence and back again. Because functional decline in older adults has similar features, current interventions used for prevention in older adults may hold promise for those in middle age. In this study, sedentary people in their middle ages were at greater risk of developing a functional impairment. Regular exercise and, if needed, weight loss may help manage medical conditions like arthritis and T2D and possibly cut the risk for future disabilities [36].

A healthy environment is also of crucial importance for the potential health benefits of walking and out-door exercise, especially in chronically ill, but also in healthy people. Short-term exposure to traffic pollution prevents the beneficial cardiopulmonary effects of walking in people with chronic obstructive pulmonary disease (COPD), ischemic heart disease, and those free from chronic cardiopulmonary diseases. Medication use might reduce the adverse effects of air pollution in individuals with ischemic heart disease. Policies should aim to control ambient levels of air pollution along busy streets in view of these negative health effects [37].

Coming to nutrition, significant declines in sugar-sweetened beverages (SSB) were observed 1 year after taxing SSBs, even in a relatively affluent community as in Berkeley, California, USA, with a general lower intake of SSBs compared to national levels. This wanted nutritional change was accompanied by revenues from public tax, potentially used for other prevention interventions. Yet, further evaluation of taxation of SSBs is needed to assess broader dietary and potential health impacts [38]. This assumption however, seems promising, since recent evidence suggests that SSB consumption is positively associated with or has an effect on obesity indices in children and adults supporting public health policies to reduce the consumption of SSBs and encourage healthy alternatives as water [39].

Also regular use of nutrition labels may have important long-term health implications. During a follow-up from 2002 and 2013, a statistical analysis suggested that in nutrition label users, the hazard risk (HR) of a diabetes diagnosis decreased significantly with time compared with the risk in nutrition label non-users. However, additional longitudinal research with a robust dietary intake analysis is needed to test this hypothesis [40].

References

1. International Diabetes Federation. IDF Diabetes Atlas 8th Edition. Available at: http://www.diabetesatlas.org/. Accessed 27 Dec 2017
2. Roeckl S, Brinks R, Baumert J et al (2017) All cause mortality in adults with and without type 2 diabetes: findings from the national health monitoring in Germany. BMJ Open Diab Res Care 5:e000451. https://doi.org/10.1136/bmjdrc-2017-000451
3. Bierman AS, Tinetti ME (2016) Precision medicine to precision care: managing multimorbidity. Lancet 388:2721–2723
4. American Diabetes Association (ADA) (2018) Prevention or delay of type 2 diabetes: standards of medical care in diabetes—2018. Diabetes Care 41(Suppl 1):S51–S54. https://doi.org/10.2337/dc18-S005
5. American Diabetes Association (ADA) (2018) Approaches to glycemic treatment: standards of medical care in diabetes—2018. Diabetes Care 41(Suppl 1):S73–S85. https://doi.org/10.2337/dc18-S008
6. Feldman AL, Griffin SJ, Al A et al (2017) Impact of weight maintenance and loss on diabetes risk and burden: a population-based study in 33,184 participants. BMC Public Health 17:170. https://doi.org/10.1186/s12889-017-4081-6
7. The Global BMI Mortality Collaboration (2016) Body-mass index and all-cause mortality: individual-participant-data-meta-analysis of 239 prospective studies in four continents. Lancet 388:776–786

8. Gao F, Wang J, Shen H et al (2018) Impact of obesity on mortality in patients with diabetes: meta-analysis of 20 studies including 250,016 patients. J Diabetes Investig 9:44–54. https://doi.org/10.1111/jdi.12677
9. Lee EY, Lee Y-h, Yi S-W, Shin S-A, Yi J-J (2017) BMI and all-cause mortality in normoglycemia, impaired fasting glucose, newly diagnosed diabetes, and prevalent diabetes: a cohort study. Diabetes Care 40:1026–1033
10. American Diabetes Association (ADA) (2018) Classification and diagnosis of diabetes: standards of medical care in diabetes—2018. Diabetes Care 41(Suppl 1):S13–S27. https://doi.org/10.2337/dc18-S002
11. Barry E, Roberts S, Oke J et al (2017) Efficacy and effectiveness of screen and treat policies in prevention of type 2 diabetes: systematic review and meta-analyis of screening tests and interventions. BMJ 356:i6538. https://doi.org/10.1136/bmj.i6538
12. Lean MEJ, Leslie WS, Barnes AC et al (2018) Primary care-led weight management for remission of T2D (direct): an open label, cluster-randomised trial. Lancet 391(10120):541–551. https://doi.org/10.1016/S0140-6736(17)33102-1
13. Tuomilehto J, Lindstrom J, Eriksson JG et al (2001) Prevention of T2D mellitus by changes in lifestyle among subjects with impaired glucose tolerance. N Engl J Med 344:1343–1350
14. Knowler WC, Barrett-Connor E, Fowler SE et al (2002) Reduction in the incidence of type diabetes with lifestyle intervention or metformin. N Engl J Med 346:393–403
15. Aroda VR, Knowler WC, Crandall JP et al (2017) For the diabetes prevention program research group. Metformin for diabetes prevention: insights gained from the diabetes prevention program/diabetes prevention program outcomes study. Diabetologia 60:1601–1611
16. Le Roux CW, Astrup A, Fujioka K et al (2017) 3 years of liraglutide vs. placebo for T2Drisk reduction and weight management in individuals with prediabetes: a randomized, double-blind trial. Lancet 389:1399–1409
17. Haw JS, Galaviz KI, Straus AN et al (2017) Long-term sustainability of diabetes prevention approaches. A systematic review and meta-analysis of randomized clinical trials. JAMA Intern Med 177:1808–1817. https://doi.org/10.1001/jamainternmed.2017.6040
18. Canpbell JM, Bellman SM, Stephensen MD et al (2017) Metformin reduces all-cause mortality and diseases independent of its effect on diabetes control: a systematic review and meta-analysis. Ageing Res Rev 40:31–44. https://doi.org/10.1016/j.arr.2017.08.003
19. Valencia WM, Palacio A, Tamariz L, Florez H (2017) Metformin and ageing: improving outcomes beyond glycaemic control. Diabetologia 60:1630–1638
20. Aroda VR, Edelstein SL, Goldberg RB et al (2016) Long-term metformin use and vitamin B12 deficiency in the diabetes prevention program outcomes study. J Clin Endocrinol Metab 101:1754–1761
21. Ocampo Chaparro JM (2013) Vitamin B12 deficit and development of geriatric syndromes. Colomb Med (Cali) 44:42–45e PMCID: PMC4002007
22. Brakedal B, Flones I, Reiter SF et al (2017) Glitazone use associated with reduced risk of Parkinson's disease. Mov Disord 32(11):1594–1599. https://doi.org/10.1002/mds.27128
23. Athauda D, Maclagan K, Skene SS et al (2017) Exenatide once weekly versus placebo in Parkinson's disease: a randomized, double-blind, plazebo-controlled trial. Lancet 390:1664–1675
24. Bae JP, Lage MJ, Mod NDR, Hoogwerf BJ (2016) Obesity and glycemic control in patients with diabetes mellitus: analysis of physician electronic health records in the US from 2009-2011. J Diab Compl 30:212–220
25. Gummesson A, Nyman E, Knutsson M, Karpefors M (2017) Effect of weight reduction on hemoglobin A1c in weight loss trials of T2D patients. Diab Obes Metab 19:1295–1305. https://doi.org/10.1111/dom.12971
26. Schauer PR, Deepak BL, Kirwan JP et al (2017) Bariatric surgery versus intensive medical therapy for diabetes—5-year outcomes. N Engl J Med 376:641–651
27. Fougere B, Morley JE (2017) Weight loss is a major cause of frailty (editorial). J Nutr Health Aging 21(9):933–935

28. Sinclair AJ, Abdelhafiz A, Dunning T et al (2017) On behalf of the expert working group. An international position statement on the management of frailty in diabetes mellitus: summary of recommendations 2017. J Frailty Aging. Available at: http://www.jfrailtyaging.com/all-issue.html?artcle=609
29. Morley JE, Anker SD (2017) Myopenia and precision (P4) medicine. J Cachexia Sarcopenia Muscle 8:857. https://doi.org/10.1002/jcsm.12231
30. Holst C, Becker U, Jorgensen ME et al (2017) Alcohol drinking patterns and risk of diabetes: a cohort study of 70,551 men and women from the general Danish population. Diabetologia 60:1941–1950. https://doi.org/10.1007/s00125-017-4359-3
31. Kondapally R, Seshasai S, Thompson A et al (2011) Diabetes mellitus, fasting glucose, and risk of cause-specific death. N Engl J Med 364:829–841
32. Schernthaner G, Lehmann R, Prazny M et al (2017) Translating recent results from the cardiovascular outcome trials into clinical practice: recommendations from the Central and Eastern European Diabetes Expert Group (CEEDEG). Cardiovasc Diabetol 16:137–149. https://doi.org/10.1186/s12933-017-0622-7
33. Currie CJ, Holden SE, Jenkins-Jones S et al (2018) Impact of differing glucose-lowering regimens on the pattern of association between glucose control and survival. J Diab Obes Metab 20:821. https://doi.org/10.1111/dom.13155
34. Sattar N, Preiss D, Murray HM et al (2010) Statins and risk of incident diabetes: a collaborative meta-analysis of randomised statin trials. Lancet 375:735–742
35. Jones M, Tett S, Peeters GMEE et al (2017) New-onset diabetes after statin exposure in elderly women: the Australian Longitudinal Study on Women's Health. Drugs Aging 34:203–209. https://doi.org/10.1007/s40266-017-0435-0
36. Brown RT, Diaz-Ramirez LG, Boscardin WJ et al (2017) Functional impairment and decline in middle age: a cohort study. Ann Intern Med 167:761–768. https://doi.org/10.7326/M17-0496
37. Sinharay R, Gong J, Barratt B et al (2018) Respiratory and cardiovascular responses to walking down a traffic-polluted road compared with walking in a traffic-free area in participants aged 60 years and older with chronic lung or heart disease and age-matched healthy controls: a randomised, cross-over study. Lancet 391:339–349. https://doi.org/10.1016/s0140-6736(17)32643-0
38. Silver LD, Ng SW, Ryan-Ibarra S, Smith Taillie L et al (2017) Changes in prices, sales, consumer spending, and beverage consumption one year after tax on sugar-sweetened beverages in Berkeley, California, US: a before-and-after study. PLoS Med 14:e1002283. https://doi.org/10.1371/journal.pmed.1002283
39. Luger M, Lafontan M, Bes-Rastrollo M et al (2017) Sugar-sweetened beverages and weight gain in children and adults: a systematic review from 2013 to 2015 and a comparison with previous studies. Obes Facts 10:674–693. https://doi.org/10.1159/000484566
40. Kollannoor-Samuel G, Shbl FM, Hawley NL, Perez-Escamilla R (2017) Nutrition label use is associated with lower long-term diabetes risk in US adults. Am J Clin Nutr 105:1079–1085. https://doi.org/10.3945/ajcn.116.145359

Life Time Prevention of Chronic Airway Diseases

9

Maciej Chałubiński and Marek L. Kowalski

Key Messages

- Asthma and chronic obstructive pulmonary disease (COPD) have been considered to be major causes of morbidity from childhood to old age.
- Prevalence of bronchial asthma reaches approximately 12% of children, 11% of adults, and 6–10% in elders. Asthma results from complex gene-environmental interactions and may have both allergic and non-allergic etiology.
- Chronic obstructive pulmonary disease (COPD) affects 10% of adult population and is the most common among elderly subjects. COPD is the fourth leading cause of death in the world.
- Although bronchial asthma and COPD result in the airway obstruction and give similar respiratory symptoms, they are separate entities with different etiology. Bronchial asthma usually develops in childhood and is associated with allergy, while COPD is associated with smoking and affects mostly adult or elderly subjects.
- A history of asthma in a childhood significantly increases the risk of chronic obstructive pulmonary disease later in life; in a proportion of patients, symptoms of asthma and COPD may co-exist, which has been referred to as the asthma COPD overlap syndrome (ACOS).
- Primary and secondary prevention of these diseases are essential and effective, "saving" age-related respiratory function decline.

M. Chałubiński · M. L. Kowalski (✉)
Department of Immunology and Allergy, Healthy Ageing Research Center (HARC), Medical University of Lodz, Łódź, Poland
e-mail: Marek.Kowalski@csk.umed.lodz.pl

J.-P. Michel (ed.), *Prevention of Chronic Diseases and Age-Related Disability*, Practical Issues in Geriatrics, https://doi.org/10.1007/978-3-319-96529-1_9

9.1 Introduction

The prevalence of chronic airway diseases has been steadily increasing in recent decades. Bronchial asthma affects 300 million individuals worldwide [1] and in the USA approximately 11% of adults and 12% of children have been diagnosed with asthma in their lifetime [2]. In Europe, asthma prevalence varies depending on the country economic status and ranges from 1.6% in Romania, 2% in Bulgaria, 5.4% in Poland, 6.7% in Spain, 7.9% in Germany, 10.6% in France to 17.8% in the UK, and 20.6% in Sweden [3]. Although asthma is among the most frequent chronic conditions in childhood, it also affects adults and elderly patients. In high income countries, the prevalence of asthma in adults above 64 years old ranges between 6 and 10%. Due to a predicted 100% increase of population aged >64 years in the next 20 years, it is reasonable to expect increasing asthma morbidity, especially that in the elderly patients asthma is often misdiagnosed, and the mortality rate remains high [4, 5].

Chronic Obstructive Pulmonary Disease (COPD) affects 10% of adult population, and is the most common among elderly subjects. In 2012, more than three million people died of COPD which is the fourth leading cause of death in the world [6]. Interestingly, in a proportion of patients, symptoms of asthma and COPD may co-exist, which has been referred to as the Asthma COPD Overlap Syndrome (ACOS). The burden of concomitant asthma and COPD is significant, given the reported overlap rate of 40–60% in elderly subjects [5].

9.2 Asthma Risk Factors

Asthma results from complex gene-environmental interactions and may have both allergic and non-allergic etiology. Multiple genes may contribute to asthma development at various ages including those related to immune response to pathogens and atopy, which is associated with tendency to synthesis of allergen-specific IgE, impaired relation between Th1- and Th2-type immune responses and bronchial hyperresponsiveness [7, 8]. Recently, particular attention has been paid to the airway epithelial integrity related to impaired tight junction functions [9]. Furthermore, differences in the prevalence of asthma between males and females suggest the importance of hormones and age; in childhood, boys are at 2 times higher risk of asthma development than girls, while in adulthood, more women suffer from asthma [7]. Additionally, in adult women, obesity becomes a relevant asthma risk factor, which is related to the late-onset of the disease.

The rapid increase of respiratory allergies and asthma prevalence may result from the influence of environmental factors on the immune system, airways and whole organism, together called an exposome. The exposome consists of 3 types of exposures: firstly, the general external environment (climate, air pollution, urban-rural residence, social capital, and education); secondly, one's specific external environment and behaviors (diet, physical activity, tobacco smoking, infection, and occupation); and, finally, the internal environment, including the biological and metabolic/toxicological manifestations of these exposures in the body [10, 11]. Respiratory tracts are particularly susceptible to air pollution from 2 key sources: (1) traffic-related air pollution (TRAP), including carbon monoxide, nitrogen oxides, benzene, ultrafine particles, and endocrine disruptors, and (2) environmental tobacco smoke. They all may affect allergic airway disease development [7, 11]. One should also consider that people working on farms, in laboratory animal facilities, painters, cleaners, and plastic manufacturers are at higher risk of asthma development [7]. Additionally, infections to human rhinovirus (HRV) and respiratory syncytial virus (RSV) in early childhood were shown to predict the allergic sensitization and the development of asthma childhood and adulthood, while CMV infection may be associated with asthma at older ages [7, 8, 12].

In a proportion of patients with asthma, allergic sensitization is not detectable; therefore, these patients are considered to have a non-allergic asthma. Etiology of this form of asthma is less clear although a pathophysiology seems to be similar, involving development of predominantly Th2-type inflammation in the airway mucosa, viral infections, and environmental factors mentioned above.

9.2.1 Asthma Primary Prevention

Strategies for asthma prevention are based on the influence on life span risk factors and include efforts associated with both primary and secondary prevention. However, limited information is available addressing primary prevention of asthma, especially with respect to allergic sensitization, and majority of studies give conflicting results. Although some studies suggested that maternal intake of food allergens may be associated with a decrease in asthma in the offspring [7], there is no firm evidence that exposure to specific foods during pregnancy decreases the risk for asthma [13]. Breast-feeding may decrease wheezing episodes in early life, but it does not seem to prevent development of persistent asthma. Similarly, maternal vitamin D and vitamin E intake was associated with lower risk of wheezing episodes in children and the development of asthma and allergic rhinitis by some studies, but not by the others [7, 14]. It is worth mentioning that antibiotics and paracetamol use by pregnant mothers and infants may also be associated with asthma development [7]. Eventually, no dietary changes during pregnancy and early maternity are recommended for prevention of allergy and asthma (Table 9.1).

There may exist a nonlinear dose–response relationship between house dust mite exposure and development of allergic disease, as exposure to both very low and very

Table 9.1 Current recommendations for asthma primary prevention, based on high quality evidence or consensus (GINA 2017 [7])

*Children should not be exposed to environmental tobacco smoke during pregnancy and after birth
*Vaginal delivery should be encouraged where possible
*Breast-feeding is advised, for reasons other than prevention of allergy and asthma
*The use of broad-spectrum antibiotics during the first year of life should be discouraged

high levels of allergen correlates with decreased risk of sensitization and asthma; while exposure to intermediate levels of allergen is associated with increased risk [10]. Similarly, exposure to pets may be associated with both increased and decreased risk of sensitization and asthma development. Some authors suggest that presence of cats or dogs during pregnancy or early childhood may exert a protective effect against hypersensitivity to these animal allergens. It is even suggested that the number of animals in the yard or at home can make a difference for the immune tolerance induction and the risk of allergic sensitization [7, 15]. Nevertheless, guidelines on allergy prevention do not recommend any measures for the house dust mite or animal allergen exposure as primary prevention (Fig. 9.1).

Prenatal, postnatal, and early-life exposure to cigarette smoke and air pollutants are of particular interest in efforts to prevent detrimental effects on lung development, as many studies have demonstrated an association between early-life exposure to pollutants and asthma. Exposure to tobacco smoke has been identified as a major risk factor for asthma, especially with in utero or during early life [16]. Increasing exposure to NO2, PM2.5, and black carbon at the birth address and

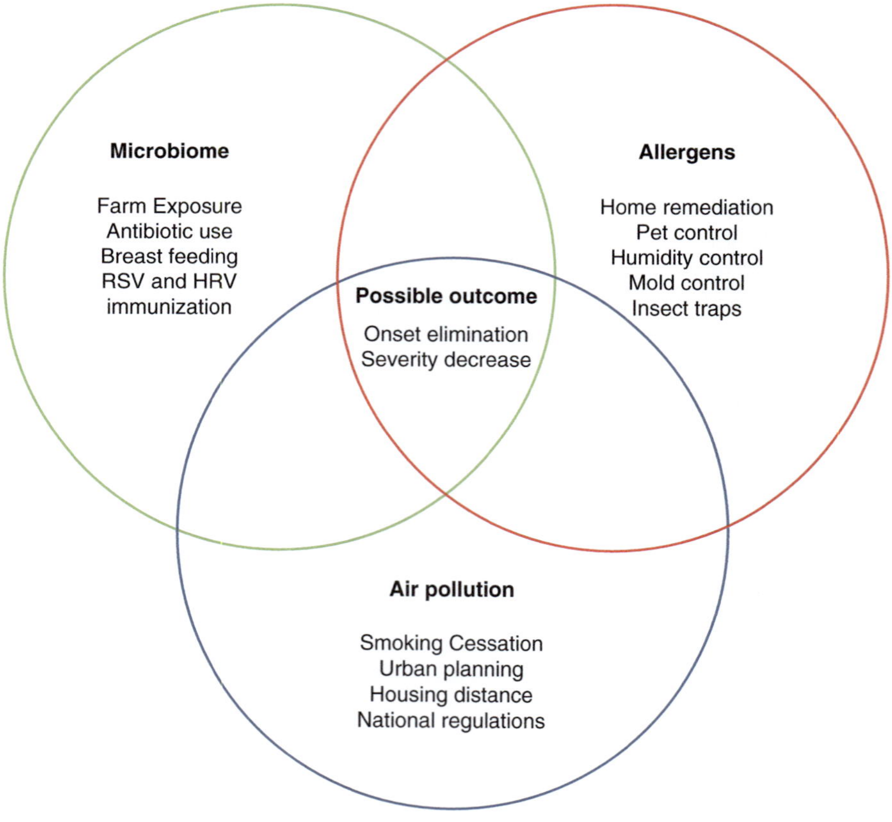

Fig. 9.1 Potential interventions reducing the risk of allergic disease development (based on [10])

childhood was shown to be associated with increased asthma incidence through adolescence [17]. Therefore, smoking cessation and avoidance of the exposure to passive smoking, and indoor and outdoor air pollutants, and conditions that promote mold are strongly recommended.

According to microflora hypothesis, the impact of microbiota on human may be beneficial in asthma prevention. Children raised on farms exposed to stables, consuming raw, unpasteurized milk, and having more bacterial-derived lipopolysaccharide endotoxin (LPS) in their bedrooms have lower risk of asthma than children of non-farmers [18]. This putative protective effect of the farming environment against childhood asthma has been attributed to the hygiene hypothesis, according to which the reduced intensity and diversity of microbial exposure is considered a major factor driving abnormal postnatal immune maturation [19]. It is believed that the influence of microbes and infections during early childhood may lead to the establishment of specific immune tolerance to allergens, thus reducing the risk of allergy and asthma development [7]. To support this approach, recent meta-analysis of 17 trials indicated that combined pre- and postnatal probiotic treatment reduced the risk of sensitization [20]. However, international expert bodies, including European Academy of Allergy and Clinical Immunology, American Academy of Pediatrics, European Society for Pediatrics Gastroenterology, Hepatology and Nutrition, National Institute of Allergy and Infectious Diseases, and WHO do not generally recommend probiotics for allergy prevention [19].

Another strategy proposed for primary prevention of asthma includes prevention of viral infection, mostly HRV and RSV, in early life. A few trials suggested lower incidence of recurrent wheezing in premature infants treated with palivizumab a monoclonal antibody against RSV, and fewer wheezing days during the first year of life. In the other study, although palivizumab decreased recurrent wheezing in up to a 6-year follow-up in preterm infants, it did not affected rates of atopic asthma [21, 22]. Whether these effects would translate into long-term prevention of asthma, still remains unknown.

9.2.2 Asthma Secondary Prevention

Secondary prevention strategies should be based mostly on the proper asthma treatment and optimal control, prevention of exacerbations due to viral and bacterial infections, and decreased exposure to aeroallergens.

One should also consider allergen-specific immunotherapy as the prevention of sensitization to aeroallergens and likelihood of asthma development. According to the concept: "one airway, one disease," asthma often co-exist with allergic rhinitis, and upper airway disease may affect asthma control and severity [7]. Allergen-specific immunotherapy in allergic rhinitis patients during their childhood and adolescence is considered a key candidate for a preventive intervention in asthma [23]. Preventive allergen therapy (PAT) study in children with seasonal allergic rhinitis demonstrated a reduction of the risk of seasonal asthma by about 50%. In the PAT study, the risk of asthma outside the pollen season was reduced in patients on pollen-specific immunotherapy, suggesting nonspecific asthma-preventing effects [23].

Future studies should focus on identifying the effect of the summation of various environmental factors and epigenetic effects of these exposures. This approach can more effectively identify the interventions that will have the greatest effect [10].

9.3 Chronic Obstructive Pulmonary Disease

Chronic Obstructive Pulmonary Disease (COPD) is common, preventable, and treatable disease characterized by persistent respiratory symptoms and airflow limitation that is due to airway and/or alveolar abnormalities usually caused by significant exposure to noxious particles or gases [6]. The most common respiratory symptoms include dyspnea, cough, and/or sputum production.

9.3.1 COPD Risk Factors

Tobacco smoking is the major risk factor for COPD development, and more than 75% of the COPD deaths have been attributed to smoke exposure [24]. However, exposure to other environmental factors, including air pollution and biomass fuel, as well as host factors, such as genetic determinants, abnormal airways development, and finally aging may lead to the development of COPD [6]. As exposure to risk factors is going to be continued and because of aging of the population, a COPD burden is projected to increase in coming decades.

9.3.2 Prevention of COPD

Smoking avoidance and/or quitting as early as possible have been recommended for both primary and secondary COPD prevention [24]. Why smoking cessation is so important? After attaining a maximum in young adulthood, in most individuals, lung volume remains constant for about 10 years, after which it slowly declines at about 20 mL per year in the healthy never-smoking individuals [25]. In tobacco smokers, the duration of the "plateau phase" is reduced and the decline begins earlier. Therefore, smoking cessation is essential for COPD management, leading to decrease in respiratory symptoms and hospitalizations, but also declining number of acute exacerbation and overall mortality. There is a strong evidence that the earlier the individual quits smoking, the more favorable will be the outcome of the disease [24]. For heavy smokers who may find difficulties with quitting this habit, effective support can be provided, including pharmaceutical approach, practical counseling as well as social and psychological support.

Although pharmacological treatment of COPD has been generally regarded as not affecting lung function decline, available study results contradict this general belief. Recent studies documented that combination of inhaled corticosteroid with long or ultra-long-lasting beta2-mimetic may result in a significant improvement in the rate of FEV1 decline [26, 27]. Proper physical activity and high-quality diet also play important roles in delaying disease process, improving quality of life, and reducing COPD-related outcomes. Therefore, adoption of healthy lifestyle behaviors, including regular exercise, and healthy diet are recommended for the self-management and secondary prevention of COPD. Additional reduction of the risk from indoor and outdoor air pollution is feasible but requires individual approaches including combination of public policy, local and national resources, and cultural changes [6].

9.4 Preventing Airway Obstruction in Childhood May Prevent Development of the Airway Disease Later in Life

Although bronchial asthma and COPD result in the airway obstruction and give similar respiratory symptoms, they both have been considered completely separate entities with different etiology. Bronchial asthma usually develops in childhood and is associated with allergy, while COPD is associated with smoking and affects mostly adult or elderly subjects. However, recent studies suggest that both obstructive airway diseases may be strongly linked together. A history of asthma in a childhood significantly increases the risk of chronic obstructive pulmonary disease later in life. Children with reduced maximum growth of FEV1 in early adulthood are at risk for early or more severe COPD [28]. Reduced lung function associated with childhood asthma, which starts in infancy may persist through childhood and adulthood, and lead to development of COPD [29]. These observations suggest that early prevention and treatment of asthma allowing for "saving" respiratory function decline may lead to better respiratory health in the adulthood and in the elderly. However, direct evidence for such effects is lacking; therefore, more prospective studies are needed to develop effective strategies allowing for lifetime prevention of chronic airway diseases.

References

1. Graham LM, Eid N (2015) The impact of asthma exacerbations and preventive strategies. Curr Med Res Opin 31:825–835
2. Griswold SK, Nordstrom CR, Clark S et al (2005) Asthma exacerbations in North American adults: who are the "frequent fliers" in the emergency department? Chest 127:1579–1586
3. https://www.erswhitebook.org/chapters/adult-asthma/
4. Gibson PG, McDonald VM, Marks GB (2010) Asthma in older adults. Lancet 376:803–813
5. Milanese M, Di Marco F, Corsico AG et al (2014) Asthma control in elderly asthmatics. An Italian observational study. Respir Med 108:1091–1099
6. Global Strategy for the Diagnosis (2017) Management, and prevention of chronic obstructive pulmonary disease. Global initiative for chronic obstructive lung disease
7. Global Strategy for Asthma Management and Prevention. Global Initiative for Asthma, 2017
8. Chinnaswamy S, Wardzynska A, Pawelczyk M et al (2017) A functional IFN-lambda4-generating DNA polymorphism could protect older asthmatic women from aeroallergen sensitization and associate with clinical features of asthma. Sci Rep 7:10500

9. Steelant B, Farre R, Wawrzyniak P et al (2016) Impaired barrier function in patients with house dust mite-induced allergic rhinitis is accompanied by decreased occludin and zonula occludens-1 expression. J Allergy Clin Immunol 137:1043–1053 e5
10. Burbank AJ, Sood AK, Kesic MJ et al (2017) Environmental determinants of allergy and asthma in early life. J Allergy Clin Immunol 140:1–12
11. Chalubinski M, Kowalski ML (2006) Endocrine disrupters—potential modulators of the immune system and allergic response. Allergy 61:1326–1335
12. Kowalski ML, Wardzynska A, Studzinska M et al (2017) Cytomegalovirus DNA is highly prevalent in the blood of patients with asthma and is associated with age and asthma traits. Allergy 72:2035–2038
13. Bunyavanich S, Rifas-Shiman SL, Platts-Mills TA et al (2014) Peanut, milk, and wheat intake during pregnancy is associated with reduced allergy and asthma in children. J Allergy Clin Immunol 133:1373–1382
14. Yepes-Nunez JJ, Brozek JL, Fiocchi A et al (2018) Vitamin D supplementation in primary allergy prevention: systematic review of randomized and non-randomized studies. Allergy 73:37–49
15. Takkouche B, Gonzalez-Barcala FJ, Etminan M et al (2008) Exposure to furry pets and the risk of asthma and allergic rhinitis: a meta-analysis. Allergy 63:857–864
16. Burke H, Leonardi-Bee J, Hashim A et al (2012) Prenatal and passive smoke exposure and incidence of asthma and wheeze: systematic review and meta-analysis. Pediatrics 129:735–744
17. Gehring U, Wijga AH, Hoek G et al (2015) Exposure to air pollution and development of asthma and rhinoconjunctivitis throughout childhood and adolescence: a population-based birth cohort study. Lancet Respir Med 3:933–942
18. House JS, Wyss AB, Hoppin JA et al (2017) Early-life farm exposures and adult asthma and atopy in the agricultural lung health study. J Allergy Clin Immunol 140:249–256 e14
19. Forsberg A, West CE, Prescott SL et al (2016) Pre- and probiotics for allergy prevention: time to revisit recommendations? Clin Exp Allergy 46:1506–1521
20. Zhang GQ, Hu HJ, Liu CY et al (2016) Probiotics for prevention of atopy and food hypersensitivity in early childhood: a PRISMA-compliant systematic review and meta-analysis of randomized controlled trials. Medicine (Baltimore) 95:e2562
21. Mochizuki H, Kusuda S, Okada K et al (2017) Palivizumab prophylaxis in preterm infants and subsequent recurrent wheezing. Six-year follow-up study. Am J Respir Crit Care Med 196:29–38
22. Jartti T, Gern JE (2017) Role of viral infections in the development and exacerbation of asthma in children. J Allergy Clin Immunol 140:895–906
23. Wahn U (2017) Preventing new sensitization and asthma onset by allergen immunotherapy: the current evidence. Curr Opin Allergy Clin Immunol 17:443–446
24. Agusti A, Celli B (2017) Natural history of COPD: gaps and opportunities. ERJ Open Res 3:00117
25. Kohansal R, Martinez-Camblor P, Agusti A et al (2009) The natural history of chronic airflow obstruction revisited: an analysis of the Framingham offspring cohort. Am J Respir Crit Care Med 180:3–10
26. Calverley PM, Anderson JA, Celli B et al (2007) Salmeterol and fluticasone propionate and survival in chronic obstructive pulmonary disease. N Engl J Med 356:775–789
27. Vestbo J, Anderson JA, Brook RD et al (2017) Fluticasone furoate and vilanterol and survival in chronic obstructive pulmonary disease with heightened cardiovascular risk (SUMMIT): a double-blind randomised controlled trial. Lancet 387:1817–1826
28. McGeachie MJ (2017) Childhood asthma is a risk factor for the development of chronic obstructive pulmonary disease. Curr Opin Allergy Clin Immunol 17:104–109
29. Bui DS, Burgess JA, Lowe AJ et al (2017) Childhood lung function predicts adult chronic obstructive pulmonary disease and asthma-chronic obstructive pulmonary disease overlap syndrome. Am J Respir Crit Care Med 196:39–46

Updated Technology and Early Detection of Cancers: Pulmonary, Breast, Colon, and Prostate

10

Fabrice Denis

Key Messages

- Recent advances in technology provide a solution in the form of patient-reported outcomes (PROs) recorded electronically using simple but methodologically robust questionnaires, completed by patients and regularly transmitted to the medical team.
- Some web-applications for patient's-reported outcome allowing relapse detection in patients who have been treated for cancer recently showed interesting survival in a multicenter randomized trial in lung cancer.
- Several institutions have successfully integrated systematic patient's-reported outcome collection into routine clinical care for relapse of various cancers but also auto-immune disease, chronic kidney, or heart failure.
- Another possible application is the early detection of cancer in high risk patients (especially smokers).
- Limitations of e-Health technology in cancer prevention are the limited use of online portals by patients, reimbursement issues, changes in the health care team dynamic. However, this technology increases both the survival and quality of life of cancer patients.

10.1 Background

Early detection of cancer or cancer relapse is an important issue to improve survival. However, up to now, one of the most common strategies to early detect cancer or for a routine follow-up after cancer treatment is to track the appearance of tumors by performing regular clinical assessments with (or without) imaging at a few months

F. Denis
Institut Inter-régional de Cancérologie Jean Bernard, Le Mans, France
e-mail: f.denis@cjb72.org

J.-P. Michel (ed.), *Prevention of Chronic Diseases and Age-Related Disability*, Practical Issues in Geriatrics, https://doi.org/10.1007/978-3-319-96529-1_10

or years of interval. Nevertheless, such a follow-up is not always without any risk since, for instance, patients with non-Hodgkin's lymphoma who received more than 8 CT scans have a probability for secondary primary malignancies twice greater than those who received less than 8 [1].

E-health applications are increasingly used by patients and physicians to monitor weight loss, blood pressure, or diabetes. The use of medical web-applications in oncology and studies on their potential clinical benefit are recent. The non-personalized approach of the follow-up after a cancer treatment is a source of anxiety for patients, which can last for several weeks before the planned imaging. Moreover, routine follow-up can delay diagnosis and treatment if recurrence occurs between planned visits. Additionally, numerous sequential imaging is expensive and has low yield in detecting asymptomatic recurrence [2, 3].

In lung cancer, which killed 1.5 millions of patients each year worldwide, at least 75% of lung cancer relapses are symptomatic and some symptoms have prognostic value in determining the clinical course and survival, patient self-reported symptoms have recently received a growing interest in oncology for their potential to improve the efficiency of follow-up and of clinical care [4–7].

10.2 Patient's-Reported Outcome

Recent advances in technology provide a solution in the form of patient-reported outcomes recorded electronically using simple but methodologically robust questionnaires, completed by patients at, or between visits over the Internet or on a smart device, with data transmitted to the medical team.

The development of some web-applications for patient's-reported outcome allowing relapse detection in patients who have been treated for cancer recently showed interesting survival in a multicenter randomized trial. For example, a novel personalized follow-up strategy for lung cancer patients based on 12 symptoms self-scored weekly and transmitted to the oncologist via an "e-follow-up application" (e-FAP) was developed with a specific algorithm for detecting lung cancer relapse. The algorithm assessed the dynamic and the association of self-reported symptoms and triggers specific notification to physician if relapse or dangerous medical conditions are suggested. The e-FAP was thus designed to provide an individualized schedule for imaging based on patient symptoms, and to strongly reduce scheduled (and expansive) imaging.

10.3 Clinical Results

Two prospective studies have shown that this e-FAP (called Moovcare™) is highly reliable and that relapses were detected (on average) 5 weeks earlier than with routine scheduled imaging [8, 9]. A pilot study suggested a better survival rate (86.6%) at one-year in the web-application arm than in a retrospective control arm (59.1%) [10]. The first phase 3 multicenter randomized clinical trial was performed to compare the survival in lung cancer patients with a high risk of relapse or progression followed by the web-mediated follow-up versus the routine follow-up [11].

In this study, clinical follow-up in both arms included oncology visits at least every 3 months. Systematic CT scans or TEP were performed every 3 months in metastatic patients in control arm and one time a year in the web-mediated follow-up (experimental arm). In both arms, additional imaging could be performed at investigator's discretion.

In experimental arm, patients were asked to report weekly their weight (assessed on their own bathroom scale) and 11 symptoms. The day they measured their weight, patients self-assessed the severity of these symptoms by grading them from 0 (no symptom) to 3 (major symptoms) for appetite loss (anorexia), fatigue (asthenia), pain, cough, depression, and breathlessness (dyspnea). The five other symptoms were evaluated by using yes-or-no answers: "yes" was answered in case of a fever greater than 38.2 °C (measured when patient felt feverish), sudden face swelling (possible superior vena cava syndrome), an occurrence of a lump under the skin (possible subcutaneous or node metastasis), voice changing (possible mediastinal involvement) and appearance or increase of blood in sputum. The 12 items were reported weekly in an electronic form and sent immediately to the medical team after completion. Patients were able to add spontaneous comments to report other symptoms or incidents in a free text window. Any additional comment automatically triggered a web-alert to the oncologist but provider judgment was used whether to follow-up by phone call.

The dynamic analysis of the weekly self-reported symptoms automatically triggered a notification sent to the medical team by e-mail when predefined criteria were fulfilled, for example: (1) three-kilogram weight total loss over a 2-weeks period, (2) two or more grade 3 symptoms, or (3) a global score greater than 6 for at least two consecutive weeks. The item scores were sent to the oncologist and nurse in a graphical format as shown in Fig. 10.1. After algorithm notification, a nurse of the institution called the patient to check whether the web reporting was accurate; if so, the oncologist was asked to contact the patient by phone. If a relapse or some dangerous condition was suggested, a clinical visit (and, if needed, imaging) was performed within 8 days after the oncologist's phone call. The use of the e-FAP was maintained during treatment for a relapse to adjust supportive care measures and to detect further progression (Fig. 10.2).

For the first time in medicine, the primary endpoint of a e-health study was overall survival. From June 2014 to January 2016, 133 patients were enrolled. The median overall survival was 19 months in the experimental and 12 months in the control arm ($p = 0.0014$), with a hazard ratio equal to 0.325 (95% CI, 0.157–0.672; $p = 0.0025$) (Fig. 10.3). The Independent Data Monitoring Committee recommended to halt the study after the planned interim survival analysis. The performance status at first detected relapse was 0–1 for 77% of the patients in the experimental arm and for 33% of those in the control arm ($p = 0.0006$). Optimal treatment was initiated in 74% of the patients in the experimental arm and in 33% of those in the control arm ($p = 0.0008$). Six-month quality of life was also significantly better in experimental arm than in control arm. In both arms, 89% of the relapses were symptomatic. The

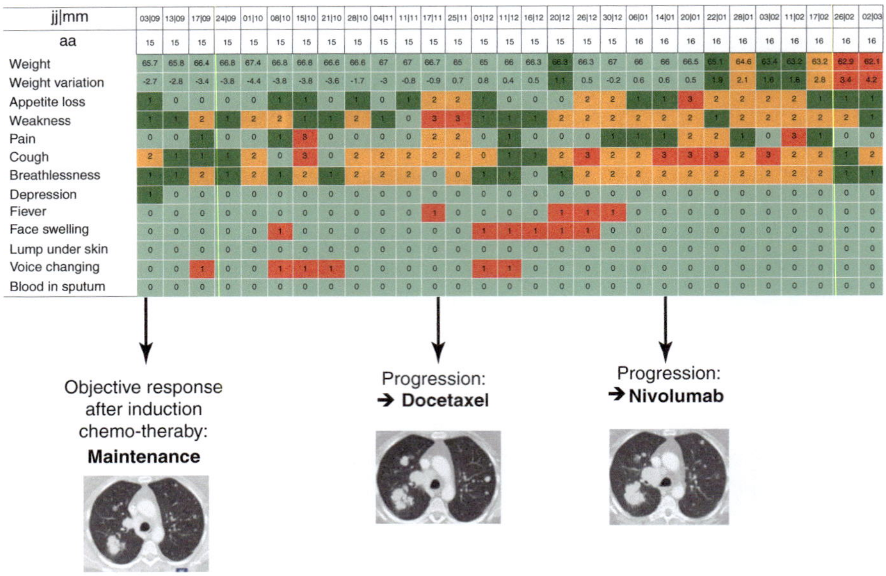

Fig. 10.1 Screenshot of the graphical representation of the evolution of a patient from his weekly completed forms. This patient had stage IV adenocarcinoma, was on maintenance therapy, and was randomized after induction chemotherapy to the experimental arm. Color legend: light green a score = 0, dark green for a score = 1, yellow for a score = 2, and red for a score = 3. In the present case, the e-FAP triggered an e-mail notification to the medical staff (see the arrow). This patient had two relapses early detected by our e-FAP (PS = 1) which were confirmed by non-scheduled imaging. A second-line chemotherapy (full dose) followed by an immunotherapy was thus initiated

relapse rate was 51% in the control arm and 49% in the experimental arm and the progression-free survivals were not significantly different between the two arms. The rate of imaging was reduced by 49%/patient/year compared to the control arm. In the experimental arm, 74% of the first relapses were detected between scheduled visits while only 33% of first relapses in the control arm were detected between visits ($p = 0.0007$). The mean duration weekly spent by the oncologist to manage all the web-alerts was 15 min for 60 simultaneous users. These results were in line with previous work utilizing electronic health initiatives. Bakitas et al. observed a greater by 15% 1-year survival improvement in cancer patients using a tele-health (phone call) follow-up right after enrollment compared to those who started the tele-health program 3 months later [12]. This study was conducted in a population with various types of cancer (lung, breast, gastrointestinal, etc.) and varying stage. Survival was not their primary outcome. A second report by Basch et al. noted an increase from 6 to 14% in the survival in 766 patients receiving chemotherapy whose symptoms were monitored via tablet computer [13]. However, this study was monocentric, in a population with various types of cancer at any stage again with survival as a secondary outcome. Moreover, the web-application allowed for monitoring the supportive care efficacy by visualization of the symptom evolution through a novel graphic This may explain the significantly higher quality of life of patients in the experimental arm at 6 months. Better quality of life could favor better survival: early management of

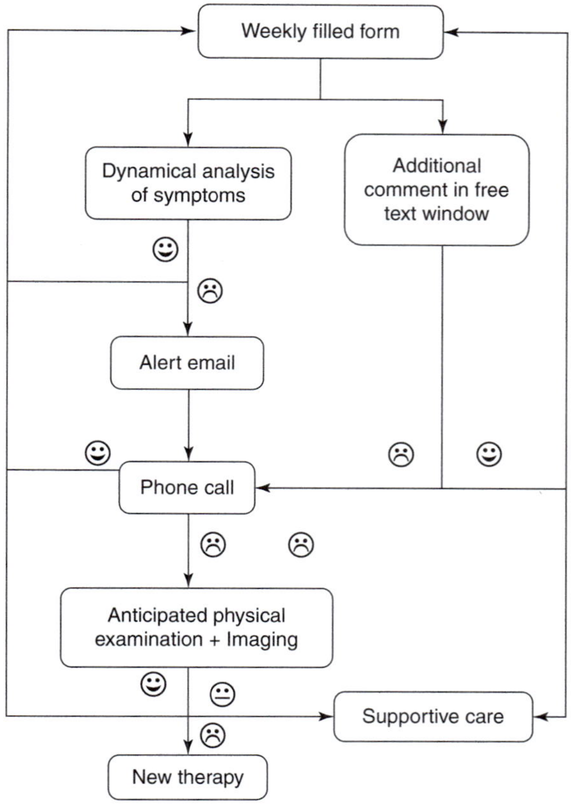

Fig. 10.2 Decision tree of the web-mediated follow-up

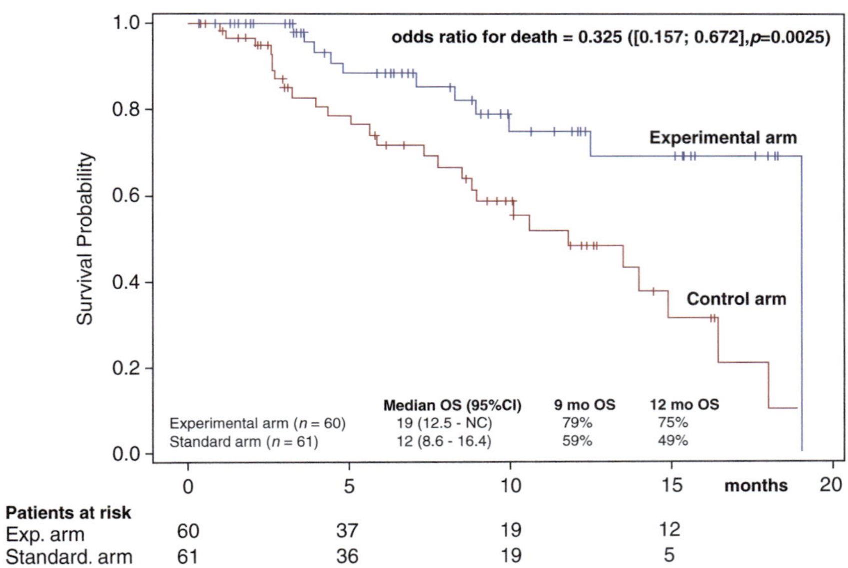

Fig. 10.3 Kaplan–Meier estimates for the survival between the initiation and the end of the trial corresponding to the planned interim analysis in Moovcare™ randomized trial [11]

physical and depressive symptoms as well as iatrogenic events may delay patient degradation, while these symptoms may be not necessarily managed as quickly with routine follow-up. Moreover, lung cancer patients are often reticent about contacting their health care providers.

Others trials in breast, colo-rectal, prostate, lymphoma, kidney cancers of web-mediated follow-up applications are in progress to assess benefit of this new modality of follow-up. There is already evidence that this approach can improve patients' quality of life, enhance patient–clinician communication, reduce emergency department use [13].

10.4 Implementation in Medical Centers

Several institutions have successfully integrated systematic patient's-reported outcome collection into routine clinical care. Since 2011, Dartmouth–Hitchcock Medical Center has collected PRO data on pain, physical functioning, and emotional health from outpatients and included them alongside vital signs in its electronic health record (EHR system), referred to as "Vitals Plus 3," for clinicians to review with patients at visits. Cincinnati Children's Hospital also began collecting PROs from outpatients with any of more than 30 chronic conditions, with information automatically loaded into EHR flow sheets to be reviewed at visits. The Cleveland Clinic systematically collects PROs from outpatients seen at 12 of its 17 disease-based institutes, an initiative that began in its Neurological Institute in 2008. This information is used for both patient care and continuous quality improvement, with data collected at more than 100,000 encounters each month. Memorial Sloan Kettering Cancer Center collects PROs from patients in several situations, including recovery from prostate and breast surgery, and feeds this information back to patients and clinicians, with graphical comparisons to similar patients. This system is being expanded to include all patients who undergo outpatient surgeries, with plans to make collection of PROs routine across all care settings [14]. In France, only the Jean Bernard Institute in Le Mans to use PRO to follow lung and prostate cancer patients since 2012 and self-developed a solution of web-mediated follow-up to early detect relapse and to improve the management of supportive cares.

10.5 Future Other Indications

Chronic diseases such as multiple sclerosis, and other auto-immune diseases, chronic kidney failure, heart failure may also benefit from this type of approach to early detect relapse as well as to improve adherence to treatment and detect toxicity.

Another approach of this follow-up could be the early detection of cancer in high risk patients. The development of an application (Smokecheck™) is in progress to detect medical complication of tobacco at first symptoms in smokers such as heart, vascular, or lung deterioration, as well as cancer. As most of lung cancers are diagnosed at an advanced stage after many months of symptoms, better prognosis may be obtain as already suggested in an evaluation of the impact of large-scale interventions to raise public awareness of a lung cancer symptom in Great Britain. In this large study, the Department of Health funded a campaign to raise public awareness of persistent cough as a lung cancer symptom and encourage people with the symptom to visit their physician. Staging, treatment, and 1-year survival was assessed [15]. There was an increase in urgent physician referrals for suspected lung cancer. The number of referrals increased by 31.8% for the campaign period. There was a 9.1% increase in lung cancers diagnosed during the campaign period (adjusted for working days; $P < 0.001$). The proportion of lung cancers diagnosed at stage I increased by 3.1 percentage points during the campaign period, (from 14.1% to 17.3%, $P < 0.001$; a proportional increase of 22%), and there was a corresponding 3.5 percentage point decrease in the proportion diagnosed at stage IV (from 52.5 to 49.0%, $P < 0.001$). A greater proportion of lung cancer patients received surgical resection as a first definitive treatment following the campaign launch (+2.3%). These encouraging results were obtained by assessing only one symptom (persistent cough). As Smokecheck™ application assessed eight more symptoms such as involuntary weight loss, blood in sputum, and dyspnea, sensitivity of lung cancer detection will be probably be improved as well as prognosis.

10.6 Limitations and Challenges

Yet examination of PROs has not become a widely implemented part of routine care delivery, which would require overcoming key barriers.

10.6.1 Technological Aspect

The most commonly used electronic health record (HER) vendors in the United States have only rudimentary ability to collect PRO data, and it's generally available only through online patient portals, which most patients don't use. PRO collection would be enabled for patients on their own smart devices in flexible user-configurable formats, perhaps through text messages, automated telephone systems, or downloadable apps. The data could then be imported into the EHR through an interface.

10.6.2 Reimbursement

Reimbursement of the PRO applications by health authorities is a major challenge to allow their deployment and their use by patients. As results of studies are encouraging and more than 1500 patients have already been included in randomized studies, reimbursement of well-assessed applications should happen soon.

10.6.3 PRO in Clinical Work-Flow

Implementation of this process required a change in the dynamics of a patient's care team by including nurses and staff, as well as a change in how patients are educated.

Other challenges are surmountable. Standards exist for ensuring data privacy and security, determining the appropriate frequency of data collection, minimizing missing data, and analyzing real-world PRO data. Concerns have been raised about burdening patients with too many questions and about patients' potential reticence about self-reporting. But research and the example implementation programs have shown that these problems are not substantial when a thoughtful approach is taken.

Conclusion

Early detection of cancer or relapse is a major challenge to improve survival. As many cancers are symptomatic and patient's reported outcome by application have demonstrated evidence of clinical relevance, patients will become full actor of their health. The improvement of communication of information between patients and physician allowed by e-health technology will become soon a standard of care at low cost.

References

1. Kahl BS, Armitage JO, Redberg R. CT use in NHL patients increase cancer risk, 19th Congress of the European Hematology 67 Association (EHA): 2014 Abstract BSSUB-3488
2. Masters GA, Temin S, Azzoli CG et al (2015) Systemic therapy for stage IV non-small-cell lung Cancer: American Society of Clinical Oncology clinical practice guideline update. J Clin Oncol 33:3488–3515
3. Meregaglia M, Cairns J (2015) Economic evaluations of follow-up strategies for cancer survivors: a systematic review and quality appraisal of the literature. Expert Rev Pharmacoecon Outcomes 15(6):913–929
4. Walsh GL, O'Connor M, Willis KM et al (1995) Is follow-up of lung cancer patients after resection medically indicated and cost-effective? Ann Thorac Surg 60:1563–1570
5. Westeel V, Choma D, Clement F et al (2000) Relevance of an intensive postoperative follow-up after surgery for non-small cell lung cancer. Ann Thorac Surg 70:1185–1190
6. Selby JV, Beal AC, Frank L (2012) The Patient-Centered Outcomes Research Institute (PCORI) national priorities for research and initial research agenda. JAMA 307:1583–1584
7. Basch E, Artz D, Dulko D et al (2005) Patient online self-reporting of toxicity symptoms during chemotherapy. J Clin Oncol 23:3552–3561
8. Denis F, Viger L, Charron A et al (2014) Detecting lung cancer relapse using self-evaluation forms weekly filled at home: the sentinel follow-up. Support Care Cancer 22:79–85
9. Denis F, Viger L, Charron A et al (2014) Detection of lung cancer relapse using self-reported symptoms transmitted via an internet web-application: pilot study of the sentinel follow-up. Support Care Cancer 22:1467–1473
10. Denis F, Yossi S, Septans AL et al (2017) Improving survival in patient treated for a lung cancer using self-evaluated symptoms reported via a web-application. Am J Clin Oncol 40(5):464–469

11. Denis F, Lethrosne C, Pourel N et al (2017) Randomized trial comparing a web-mediated follow-up to routine surveillance in lung cancer patients. J Natl Cancer Inst 109(9). https://doi.org/10.1093/jnci/djx029
12. Bakitas MA, Tosteson TD, Li Z et al (2015) Early versus delayed initiation of concurrent palliative oncology care: patient outcomes in the ENABLE III randomized controlled trial. J Clin Oncol 33:1438–1445
13. Basch E, Deal AM, Kris MG et al (2015) Symptom monitoring with patient-reported outcomes during routine cancer treatment: a randomized controlled trial. J Clin Oncol 34:557–565
14. Basch E (2017) Patient-reported outcomes—harnessing patients' voices to improve clinical care. NEJM 376:105–108
15. Ironmonger L, Ohuma E, Ormiston-Smith N et al (2015) An evaluation of the impact of large-scale interventions to raise public awareness of a lung cancer symptom. Br J Cancer 112:207–216

Mastering Osteoporosis 11

Manfred Gogol

Key Messages

1. Osteoporosis is preventable and treatable.
2. Osteoporosis is often not diagnosed.
3. Geriatric rehabilitation, orthogeriatric services, and fracture liaison services improve outcomes.
4. Osteoporosis is associated with frailty and sarcopenia.
5. Osteoporosis is a geriatric syndrome associated with functional decline, reduced quality of life, higher institutionalization rate, high comorbidity and mortality.

Osteoporosis is a systemic skeletal disorder characterized by diminished bone mass and impaired microarchitecture of the bone tissue. It is associated with reduced strength and increased fracture risk. Technically, osteoporosis is diagnosed by taking bone mineral density (BMD) measurements and is defined as a BMD of < -2.5 standard deviations (SD) below the mean score in healthy young women. By contrast, osteopenia, the precursor to osteoporosis, is defined as a BMD < -1 to -2.5 SD below the mean score of a healthy younger reference population [1]. The presence of osteoporotic fractures, especially in the vertebrae, verifies the diagnosis. Given the frequent lack of clinical symptoms, however, the absence of fractures is not a criterion for ruling out osteoporosis.

11.1 Pathophysiology

Bone tissue is actively remodelled through a coupled process of osseous formation and resorption. Women reach their peak bone mass between the age of 25 and 35 years. In simple terms, osseous tissue undergoes continuous flux of

M. Gogol
Institute of Gerontology, Heidelberg University, Heidelberg, Germany

J.-P. Michel (ed.), *Prevention of Chronic Diseases and Age-Related Disability*, Practical Issues in Geriatrics, https://doi.org/10.1007/978-3-319-96529-1_11

formation and resorption processes with increasing and decreasing bone matrix mineralization. Resorption predominates in postmenopausal women and the elderly of either sex, in particular, resulting in decreased bone mass and altered microarchitecture [2]. Basically, osteoporosis is an age-related disease of both genders: Due to postmenopausal changes, women tend to be affected earlier, more often and more severely because their peak bone mass is lower compared to that of men [3, 4].

It is remarkable that the interrelationship between bone and other organs is manifold and complex and not fully understood yet [5]. This is even true for the relationship of muscles and bones [6]. These close biological and functional interactions between bone, muscle, and connective tissue led to the recent coinage of the—albeit not yet generally accepted—term osteosarcopenia [7].

11.2 Epidemiology

With age, the incidence of osteopenia, osteoporosis, and subsequent fractures increases. As a rule of thumb, women are affected by an osteoporotic fracture two to three times as frequently as men. Manifesting in women earlier than in men, osteopenia and osteoporosis occur with an increasing frequency in association with age of both sexes. Fractures of the trabecular bones (femur, vertebrae) are primarily involved. Given the sequelae of fractures in terms of reduced functionality, increased (co-)morbidity, reduced quality of life, higher mortality, and costs burdening the social and healthcare systems, it is clear that the disease is of utmost importance for the individual patient and, in light of its socioeconomic consequences, for society as well. The International Osteoporosis Foundation estimated for the European Union approximately 22 million women and 5.5 million men having osteoporosis and prognosed an increase of 23% in 2025 compared to 2010. For 2010, the number of new fractures was estimated at 3.5 million [8].

It is important to remember that osteoporosis and fragility fractures usually happen in a context of comorbidity [9] or multimorbidity [10], especially in the context of frailty and sarcopenia [11, 12].

11.3 Fractures

Fractures secondary to falls or even under normal weight bearing are typical sequelae of osteoporosis. At the same time, this fact is clear evidence that exogenous factors are additive to the clinical sequelae [13, 14]. Osteoporosis must therefore be regarded as a systemic disease, impacted by both endogenous (e.g., muscle mass and strength) and exogenous (e.g., domestic environments increasing the propensity to fall) contexts. Especially vertebral fractures can remain clinically asymptomatic and are often diagnosed as incidental findings after the clinical examination or revealed by imaging procedures. Nevertheless, it can be difficult to distinguish between degenerative and fracture-related changes in each individual case. Unlike fractures of the upper or lower extremity, vertebral fractures may cause few symptoms. For that reason, the patient's body height should be measured by the primary care physician once a year.

Besides an elevated 30-day and 1-year mortality secondary to osteoporotic fractures [15, 16], elderly patients in particular will frequently suffer iatrogenic complications from their hospital treatment (e.g., deconditioning, e.g., delirium) [17]. They also show functional limitations involving a reduction in their ability to carry out activities of daily living (ADL) and instrumental activities on the daily living scale (IADL). This can result in the need for nursing care alongside an elevated rate of institutionalization despite any intensive rehabilitative interventions they may undergo [18]. Second only to pain, functional limitations are the central components that detract from quality of life. These are compounded by depression and anxiety about a new fall occurring in the future (fear of falling) [19]—an event that will often impair the individual's mobility even more (Fig. 11.1).

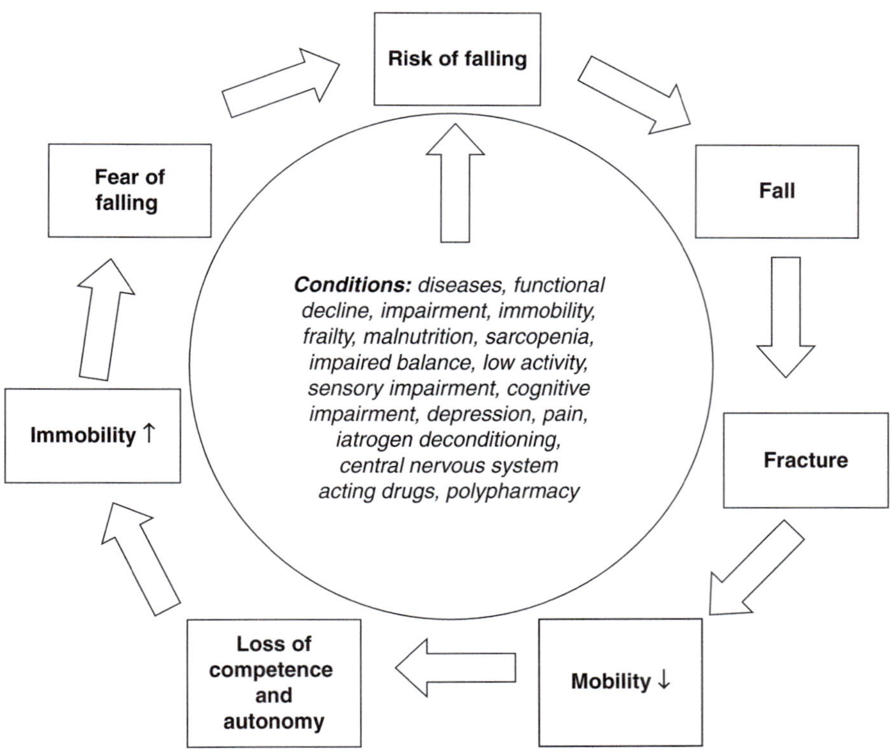

Fig. 11.1 Cycle of risk for falling/falls and consequences

11.4 Risk Factors

Risk factors can be subdivided into a category that suggests low BMD and a category that is predictively significant for fractures. In osteoporosis, risk factors associated with broken bones are particularly important. These factors can be used to identify high-risk groups and allow early initiation of preventive and/or therapeutic interventions. Osteoporosis-related fractures can be attributed to a multitude of causes. According to the current state of knowledge, unequivocal responsibility or decisive significance cannot be ascribed to any one single risk factor. Rather, a distinction should be made between constitutional, genetic, lifestyle-related, and medical risk factors. The risk factors for falls represent another group of striking importance in elderly patients. Furthermore, it is important to identify a previous fracture event as an independent and significant risk factor for further fractures [20].

Immobility in the elderly is a significant risk factor in and of itself and interrelated with muscular status, such as reductions in muscle mass, muscle strength, and overall functionality (e.g., low walking speed). It must be pointed out that social deprivation [21] and air pollution [22] are associated with a higher risk for osteoporosis and fractures.

Box 11.1 shows well-known general risk factors for osteoporosis and fractures.

Box 11.2 presents known specific risk factors for osteoporosis and fractures.

Box 11.3 shows a list of drug classes that can induce osteoporosis or propensity to fall.

Box 11.1

Age
Deficiency in specific sex hormones
Sex (women > men)
Previous fractures
Familial risk (proximal femur fracture in parents)
Genetic predisposition
Medication
Immobility
Inactivity
Balance disorders
Reduced muscle mass/strength
History of falls
Other risk factors predisposing to falls
Malnutrition
Underweight

Box 11.2

Calcium deficiency
Vitamin D deficiency
Smoking
COPD
Heart failure
Hyperhomocysteinemia
Vitamin B12 deficiency
Folic acid deficiency
Elevated hsCRP
Hyponatremia
Cushing's disease
- Subclinical hypercortisolism

Primary hyperparathyroidism
Growth hormone deficiency
Subclinical and manifest hyperthyroidism
Diabetes mellitus (I > II)
Rheumatoid arthritis
Ankylosing spondylitis
Gastrectomy, total or Billroth II
Epilepsy
Celiac disease
Monoclonal gammopathy

Box 11.3

Osteoporosis-inducing drugs
Glucocorticoids
Hormonal ablative therapy
Aromatase inhibitors
Glitazones
Proton pump inhibitors
Bisphosphonates
Elevate propensity to fall
Sedatives
Hypnotics
Neuroleptics
Antidepressants
Loop diuretics
All antihypertensives at too-high doses

11.5 Diagnostics

Alongside targeted medical history-taking, documentation of potential risk factors and the clinical findings, DEXA is the diagnostic method of choice [23]. DEXA is preferably performed on the femur or lumbar spine and shows very high accuracy in measuring BMD. Other technical measurements compromise quantitative ultrasound and variety of computer tomographic techniques, but are only to be considered as second-line diagnostics [24].

Given the association between fractures and falls, elderly patients aged 70 years and older should undergo a geriatric assessment of their fall risk in order to be able to initiate preventive interventions in a targeted manner [25]. Such measures especially involve nutritional counselling/interventions, physical training regimens, etc.

The baseline tests performed by the clinical laboratory cover the following parameters: blood sedimentation rate, blood count and differential blood count, serum calcium, alkaline phosphatase, creatinine, gamma-GT as well as serum electrophoresis if the patient has a high blood sedimentation rate. The measurement of vitamin D [26] is not generally recommended.

11.6 Therapy

It is essential to recognize that most intervention studies on osteoporosis didn't include very old patients [27] instead of the high prevalence even in the oldest old [28]. General therapeutic interventions also include ones that antagonize the aforementioned risk factors. Calorically sufficient and protein-adapted nutrition, a sufficient supply of calcium in the diet, supplemental doses of 800–1000 units of vitamin D per day and promoting an active lifestyle are all part of these interventions. Other targeted measures combine strength and balance training along with longer term rehabilitative interventions to manage the fracture sequelae, especially in post-fracture status. Beyond this, consultations concerning general fall prevention, assistive devices and, as appropriate, modifications to the patient's living space should all be conducted [29–31].

Medical calcium ought only to be supplemented if the patient's medical history or interventions show that a sufficient calcium supply of 1 g per day cannot be achieved through their diet. It can be assumed that individuals aged 70 years and older living in Central and Northern Europe will exhibit lowered vitamin D levels or vitamin D deficiency, especially if they have insufficient sun exposure. In this regard, it is not an absolute recommendation that vitamin D levels be determined in the serum. Nevertheless, their measurement may be indicated whenever there is any doubt about the patient's adherence or the efficacy of the selected supplement. As vitamin D and calcium supplementation is the basis of drug treatment, specific drugs are available to treat older patients with osteoporosis. The drugs are bisphosphonates, denosumab, teriparatide, estrogen hormone replacement, selective estrogen receptor modulator (SERM), and strontium ranelate [32]. Bisphosphonates are worldwide the most used agent. In the USA, calcitonin is in addition a therapeutic option.

Box 11.4 provides an overview of primary and secondary preventive interventions.

Box 11.4
Physical activity
Strength and balance training
Determine fall risk from 70th year of life
Fracture risk assessment
Adequate diet (protein-rich)
Nicotine abstinence
Compensate for vitamin D and calcium deficiency
Review drugs taken for their propensity to induce falls
Specific antiosteoporotic medication

Scoring systems and fracture assessment tools (e.g., FRAX [33, 34], QFracture [35, 36]) can be very helpful in estimating the future risk of fractures. Both tools are available free at the web [34, 36]. Often, show cards are also useful aids to support consultation and decision-making about therapy [37].

After a patient has sustained a fracture, appropriate outpatient and partially or fully hospitalized rehabilitative interventions must be initiated. Treatment rendered in specific geriatric [38, 39] or orthogeriatric departments [40] has produced superior outcomes in geriatric patients. Instead of different available therapies older patients very often receive no primary or secondary prevention for osteoporosis [41–43] and even adherence is often low [44]. Fracture liaison services set up because secondary preventive therapy is often not carried out and have proven their effectiveness in the induction of and adherence to a specific therapy [45].

Conclusion

Osteoporosis is a systemic, age-associated disease; the fractures it causes make its individual and social implications very apparent. These, in turn, are associated with elevated (co-)morbidity, functional limitations, reduced quality of life, increased rate of institutionalization, and greater mortality. Osteoporosis constitutes a condition that is frequently neither diagnosed properly nor treated effectively and efficiently, even though a broad spectrum of therapeutic options is available. Specific rehabilitative interventions (geriatric or orthogeriatric) secondary to fracture are effective. By putting fracture liaison services in place, the probability is increased that antiosteoporotic therapy will be initiated and adhered to. In light of the changing demographics, it can be expected that there will be a rise in the frequency of the clinical picture of osteoporosis, its associated fractures and their sequelae.

References

1. Kanis JA, on behalf of the World Health Organization Scientific Group (2007) Assessment of osteoporosis at the primary health-care level. World Health Organization Collaborating Centre for Metabolic Bone Diseases, University of Sheffield, UK. https://www.sheffield.ac.uk/FRAX/pdfs/WHO_Technical_Report.pdf
2. Howard GA, Schiller PC (2016) Biology of bone. In: Duque G, Kiel DP (eds) Osteoporosis in older persons—advances in pathophysiology and therapeutic approaches, 2nd edn. Springer, Basel, pp 1–42
3. Colón-Emeric CS (2016) Osteoporosis as a geriatric syndrome. In: Duque G, Kiel DP (eds) Osteoporosis in older persons—advances in pathophysiology and therapeutic approaches, 2nd edn. Springer, Basel, pp 131–140
4. Bischoff-Ferrari HA (2016) Fracture epidemiology among individuals 75+. In: Duque G, Kiel DP (eds) Osteoporosis in older persons—advances in pathophysiology and therapeutic approaches, 2nd edn. Springer, Basel, pp 157–170
5. Okamoto K, Nakashima T, Shinohara M et al (2017) Osteoimmunology: the conceptual framework unifying the immune and skeletal systems. Physiol Rev 97:1249–1349
6. Tarantino U, Piccirilli E, Fantini M et al (2015) Sarcopenia and fragility fractures: molecular and clinical evidence of the bone-muscle interaction. J Bone Joint Surg Am 97:429–437
7. Hirschfeld HP, Kinsella R, Duque G (2017) Osteosarcopenia: where bone, muscle, and fat collide. Osteoporos Int 28:2781–2790
8. Hernlund E, Svedbom A, Ivergård M et al (2013) Osteoporosis in the European Union: medical management, epidemiology and economic burden. A report prepared in collaboration with the international osteoporosis foundation (IOF) and the European Federation of Pharmaceutical Industry Associations (EFPIA). Arch Osteoporos 8:136
9. Pedersen AB, Ehrenstein V, Szépligeti SK, Sørensen HAT (2017) Hip fracture, comorbidity, and the risk of myocardial infarction and stroke: a Danish nationwide cohort study, 1995-2015. J Bone Miner Res 32(12):2339–2346. https://doi.org/10.1002/jbmr.3242
10. O'Malley CD, Tran N, Zapalowski C et al (2014) Multimorbidity in women with and without osteoporosis: results from a large US retrospective cohort study 2004-2009. Osteoporos Int 25:2117–2130
11. Cesari M, Prince M, Amuthavalli J et al (2016) Frailty: an emerging public health priority. J Am Med Dir Assoc 17:188–192
12. Martin FC (2017) Frailty, sarcopenia, falls and fractures. In: Falashi P, Marsh DR (eds) Orthogeriatrics, practical issues in geriatrics. Springer, Basel, pp 14–61
13. Mänty M, Heinonen A, Viljanen A et al (2010) Self-reported preclinical mobility limitation and fall history as predictors for future falls in older women: prospective cohort study. Osteoporos Int 21:689–693
14. Barbour KE, Lui L-Y, McCulloch CE et al (2016) Trajectories of lower extremity physical performance: effects on fractures and mortality in older women. J Gerontol A Biol Sci Med Sci 71(12):1609–1615. https://doi.org/10.1093/gerona/glw071
15. Darbá J, Kaskens L, Pérez-Álvarez N et al (2015) Disability-adjusted-life-years losses in postmenopausal women with osteoporosis. BMC Public Health 15:324
16. Roth T, Kammerlander C, Gosch M et al (2010) Outcome in geriatric fracture patients and how it can be improved. Osteoporos Int 21(Suppl 4):S615–S619
17. Pioli G, Bendini C, Pignedoli P (2017) Post-operative management. In: Falashi P, Marsh DR (eds) Orthogeriatrics, practical issues in geriatrics. Springer, Basel, pp 111–129
18. Hertz K, Santy-Tomlinson J (2017) The nursing role. In: Falashi P, Marsh DR (eds) Orthogeriatrics, practical issues in geriatrics. Springer, Basel, pp 131–144
19. Trombetti A, Reid KF, Hars M et al (2016) Age-associated declines in muscle mass, strength, power, and physical performance: impact on fear of falling and quality of life. Osteoporos Int 27:463–471

20. Schürer S, Wallaschofski H, Nauck M et al (2015) Fracture risk and risk factors for osteoporosis. Results from two representative population-based studies in north East Germany (study of health in Pomerania: SHIP-2 and SHIP-trend). Dtsch Arztebl Int 112:365–371
21. Bhimjiyani A, Neuburger J, Jones T et al (2018) The effect of social deprivation on hip fracture incidence in England has not changed over 14 years: an analysis of the English hospital episodes Statstics (2001-2015). Osteoporos Int 29(1):115–124. https://doi.org/10.1007/s00198-017-4238-2
22. Prada D, Zhong J, Colicino E et al (2017) Association of air particulate pollution with bone loss over time and bone fracture risk: analysis of data from two independent studies. Lancet Planet Health 1:e337–e347
23. Grossman J, MacLean CH (2007) Quality indicators for the care of osteoporosis in vulnerable elders. J Am Geriatr Soc 55:S392–S402
24. Kanis JA, McCloskey EV, Johansson H et al (2013) European guidance for the diagnosis and management of osteoporosis in postmenopausal women. Osteoporos Int 24:23–57
25. Ellis G, Whitehead MA, Robinson D et al (2011) Comprehensive geriatric assessment for older adults admitted to hospital: meta-analysis of randomised controlled trials. BMJ 343:d6553
26. Caillet P, Goyer-Joos A, Viprey M, Schott A-M (2017) Increase of vitamin D assays prescriptions and associated factors: population-based cohort study. Sci Rep 7:10361
27. McGarvey C, Coughlan T, O'Neill D (2017) Ageism in studies on the management on osteoporosis. J Am Geriatr Soc 65:1566–1568
28. Jopp DS, Boemer K, Rott C (2016) Health and disease at age 100—findings from the second Heidelberg centenarian study. Dtsch Artzebl Int 113:203–210
29. Reck BR, Daly RM, Fiatarone MA, Taaffe DR (2017) Exercise and sports science Australia (ESSA) position statement on exercise prescribtion for the prevention and management of osteoporosis. J Sci Med Sport 20:438–445
30. Lord SR, Close JCT, Sherrington C (2016) Non-pharmacological treatments for falls and fractures. In: Duque G, Kiel DP (eds) Osteoporosis in older persons—advances in pathophysiology and therapeutic approaches, 2nd edn. Springer, Basel, pp 187–200
31. Kastner M, Perrier L, Munce SEP et al (2018) Complex interventions can increase osteopororsis investigations and treatment: a systematic review and meta-analysis. Osteoporos Int 29(1):5–17. https://doi.org/10.1007/s00198-017-4248-0
32. Wong EK-W, Kim LH-Y, Papaioannou A (2016) Medical treatment of age related osteoporosis. In: Duque G, Kiel DP (eds) Osteoporosis in older persons—advances in pathophysiology and therapeutic approaches, 2nd edn. Springer, Basel, pp 201–214
33. Watts NB, Manson JE (2017) Osteoporosis and fracture risk evaluation and management—shared decision making in clinical practice. JAMA 317:253–254
34. https://www.sheffield.ac.uk/FRAX/
35. Dagan N, Cohen-Stavi C, Leventer-Roberts M, Balicer RD (2017) External validation and comparison of three prediction tools for risk of osteoporotic fractures using data from population based electronic health records: retrospective cohort study. BMJ 356:i6755
36. http://www.qfracture.org/
37. http://shareddecisions.mayoclinic.org/
38. Bachmann S, Finger C, Huss A et al (2010) Inpatient rehabilitation specifically designed for geriatric patients: systematic review and meta-analysis of randomised controlled trials. BMJ 340:c1718
39. Dyer S, Diong J, Crotty M, Sherrington C (2017) Rehabilitation following hip fracture. In: Falashi P, Marsh DR (eds) Orthogeriatrics, practical issues in geriatrics. Springer, Basel, pp 145–163
40. Friedman SM (2016) The orthogeriatrics model of care. In: Duque G, Kiel DP (eds) Osteoporosis in older persons—advances in pathophysiology and therapeutic approaches, 2nd edn. Springer, Basel, pp 265–273
41. Flais J, Coiffier G, Le Noach J et al (2017) Low prevalence of osteoporosis treatment in patients with recurrent major osteoporotic fracture. Arch Osteoporos 12:54

42. Gunathilake R, Epstein E, McNeill S, Walsh B (2016) Factors associated with receiving anti-osteoporosis treatment among older persons with minimal trauma hip fracture presenting to an acute orthogeriatric service. Injury 47:2149–2154
43. Liu Z, Weaver J, de Papp A et al (2016) Disparities in osteoporosis treatments. Osteoporos Int 27:509–519
44. Garcia-Sempere A, Hurtado I, Sanfélix-Genovés J et al (2017) Primary and secondary non-adherence to osteoporotic medications after hip fracture in Spain. The PREV2FO population-based study. Sci Rep 7:11784
45. Mitchell PJ (2016) Fracture liaison services. In: Duque G, Kiel DP (eds) Osteoporosis in older persons—advances in pathophysiology and therapeutic approaches, 2nd edn. Springer, Basel, pp 215–228

Remaining Debates on Osteoarthrosis Prevention

12

Nicola Veronese and Stefania Maggi

Key Messages

- The prevalence of osteoarthritis significantly varies depending on several factors, particularly the definition used (clinical, radiological, mixed, self-reported), age, gender, and geographical areas.
- The risk of developing osteoarthritis is determined by local factors (biomechanical), specific systemic risk factors (age, being women, poor nutritional status, and smoking) as well as other medical conditions which increase disability outcomes.
- Mediterranean diet, allowing weight loss and increasing micro-element intakes, is associated with a decreased prevalence of lower limbs osteoarthritis, better quality of life, and functionality.
- In people having osteoarthritis, the role of exercise is still debated, but aquatic exercises may have clinically relevant effects on patient-reported pain, disability, and quality of life.
- Quitting smoking is a necessary recommendation for people having osteoarthritis.
- However, more scientific studies are needed to better understand the physiopathology and the best possible preventive actions.

12.1 Introduction: Importance of Osteoarthritis

Osteoarthritis is a degenerative disease of the joints that, however, involves the cartilage, surrounding the tissues of the joints affected [1].

N. Veronese · S. Maggi (✉)
National Research Council, Neuroscience Institute, Aging Branch, Padova, Italy
e-mail: stefania.maggi@in.cnr.it

J.-P. Michel (ed.), *Prevention of Chronic Diseases and Age-Related Disability*, Practical Issues in Geriatrics, https://doi.org/10.1007/978-3-319-96529-1_12

Osteoarthritis may develop in any joint, but most commonly affects the knees, hips, hands, facet joints, and feet [2]. It is known that the prevalence of osteoarthritis significantly varies depending on several factors, particularly the definition used (clinical, radiological, mixed, self-reported), age, sex (in women its presence is higher), and the geographical area studied. In the European Project on OSteoArthritis (EPOSA) study, an European survey regarding the impact of osteoarthritis on several outcomes, osteoarthritis affected about one person over three [3], but, as mentioned before, largely varies according to site and diagnostic method used [4]. The incidence of hand, hip, and knee OA increases with age, and women have higher rates than men, especially after menopause [2].

The risk of developing osteoarthritis is determined by several factors and traditionally categorized in local and systemic. Local factors are commonly biomechanical (e.g., trauma) acting against the forces applied to the joint. A number of specific systemic risk factors [2] have been identified and they include obesity, age, female sex, ethnicity and race, poor nutrition, and smoking [5].

The consequences of osteoarthritis are multiplex. The most common (and important in older people) is disability [6]. However, increasing research has shown that osteoarthritis is associated with a higher risk of other medical conditions, such as cardiovascular diseases [7–11], psychiatric conditions (such as depression [9], anxiety [12], or dementia [13]), and poorer quality of life [14, 15]. Conversely, the association between osteoarthritis and mortality is still debated and seems to depend more on factors associated with osteoarthritis (particularly disability) than osteoarthritis per se [7].

Given its remarkable consequences and given that no therapy is available for treating osteoarthritis, prevention of this condition is necessary. Therefore, in this chapter, we aimed to summarize the current evidences regarding preventive strategies for osteoarthritis and lights/shadows regarding this topic.

12.2 Preventive Actions for Osteoarthritis

12.2.1 Dietary Suggestions

As mentioned before, some risk factors for osteoarthritis are nutritional, e.g., obesity and the lack of appropriate micronutrients necessary for bones, joints, and cartilages [16]. In several studies, weight loss in obese patients having osteoarthritis, improves quality of life, autonomy in daily living, and clinical aspects of osteoarthritis, particularly when osteoarthritis affects lower limbs [17]. Similarly, the deficiency of some nutrients (such as vitamin D) can play a role in the development of osteoarthritis [18]. Unfortunately, the supplementation with oral vitamin D metabolites seems not to be efficacious in improving osteoarthritis' symptomatology, as shown by some recent large trials [19]. This is the first important point of debate in the prevention of osteoarthritis since, whilst people having osteoarthritis have significant lower levels of circulating vitamin D metabolites [18], the replacement with vitamin D seems not to change the natural history of this condition [19].

In this regard, the suggestion to follow healthier diets seems to be more indicated. Mediterranean diet might be associated not only with a lower prevalence of lower limbs osteoarthritis [16], but also with a better quality of life and better function in people affected by knee osteoarthritis [15]. This is probably due to several beneficial effects of Mediterranean diet, such as lowering inflammatory parameters, promoting a decrease in body weight and giving abundant sources of vitamins and anti-oxidant nutrients [20]. Unfortunately, no interventional trials are available regarding the potential beneficial effects of Mediterranean diet on osteoarthritis in human beings, even if the observational data are encouraging.

12.2.2 Physical Activity

In people having osteoarthritis, the role of physical exercise is still debated. Since osteoarthritis, particularly when affecting the knees, can derive from traumas and physical exercise can further worse joint's structure, physical exercise should be strictly monitored in people having severe forms of knee osteoarthritis. However, in other stages, physical exercise should be recommended. A recent Cochrane review suggests that aquatic exercise (a kind of mild physical exercise) may have clinically relevant effects on patient-reported pain, disability, and quality of life in people having knee and hip osteoarthritis [21]. A short-term aerobic exercise program with/without muscle strengthening exercises seems to be promising for reducing pain, improving physical function and quality of life for individuals having knee osteoarthritis [22]. On the contrary, no definitive conclusion can be proposed regarding the use of muscle resistance training in people affected by lower limbs osteoarthritis, as reported by another recent systematic review [23]. Similarly, very limited evidence is available regarding the role of physical exercise in improving hand osteoarthritis outcomes [24]. Altogether, these results suggested that physical exercise is controversial in preventing or treating osteoarthritis, suggesting that other studies are consequently needed.

12.2.3 Smoking

Cigarette smoking is a very controversial topic regarding the prevention and the treatment of osteoarthritis. As widely known, smoking has several deleterious effects, such as on cardiovascular and cancer conditions. On the contrary, literature suggests that the association between smoking and osteoarthritis is probably inverse, i.e., smokers have a significant lower risk of having osteoarthritis. In fact, in a large meta-analysis involving 48 observational studies and 537,730 participants, there was an overall negative association between smoking and osteoarthritis, particularly when referring to case-control studies [25]. However, as proposed by the same authors, the protective effect of smoking in osteoarthritis is probably biased by the design of these studies [25]. In a large cohort study, involving American community-dwellers, cigarette smoking was not protective for the onset of knee osteoarthritis [26], suggesting, again, that quitting smoking is a necessary recommendation for people having osteoarthritis, waiting for specific literature regarding quitting smoking and prevention of osteoarthritis.

Conclusion

The prevention of osteoarthritis is a public health priority. Osteoarthritis, in fact, is one of the most important contributors of global disability in older people [27]. Whilst we have cleared the possible risk factors for osteoarthritis, the prevention of this condition is still debated and mainly related to some observational studies that, for their nature, are often biased. Thus, interventional studies having as outcome the onset of osteoarthritis are needed to see if the preventive strategies commonly used (losing weight, suggesting healthy dietary diets, promoting physical exercise, and quitting smoking) are able to decrease the onset of this important medical condition.

References

1. Kinds MB, Welsing PMJ, Vignon EP et al (2011) A systematic review of the association between radiographic and clinical osteoarthritis of hip and knee. Osteoarthr Cartil 9:768–778. https://doi.org/10.1016/j.joca.2011.01.015
2. Litwic A, Edwards MH, Dennison EM et al (2013) Epidemiology and burden of osteoarthritis. Br Med Bull 105:185–199. https://doi.org/10.1093/bmb/lds038
3. Castell MV, van der Pas S, Otero A et al (2015) Osteoarthritis and frailty in elderly individuals across six European countries: results from the European Project on OSteoArthritis (EPOSA). BMC Musculoskelet Disord 16:359. https://doi.org/10.1186/s12891-015-0807-8
4. Schaap LA, Peeters GMEE, Dennison EM et al (2011) European Project on Osteoarthritis (EPOSA): methodological challenges in harmonization of existing data from five European population-based cohorts on aging. BMC Musculoskelet Disord 12:272. https://doi.org/10.1186/1471-2474-12-272
5. Hunter DJ, Felson DT (2006) Osteoarthritis. BMJ 332:639–642. https://doi.org/10.1136/bmj.332.7542.639
6. Jordan J, Luta G, Renner J et al (1997) Knee pain and knee osteoarthritis severity in self-reported task specific disability: the Johnston County Osteoarthritis Project. J Rheumatol 24:1344–1349
7. Veronese N, Cereda E, Maggi S et al (2016) Osteoarthritis and mortality: a prospective cohort study and systematic review with meta-analysis. Semin Arthritis Rheum 46:160–167. https://doi.org/10.1016/j.semarthrit.2016.04.002
8. Veronese N, Trevisan C, De Rui M et al (2016) Association of osteoarthritis with increased risk of cardiovascular diseases in the elderly: findings from the Progetto Veneto Anziano study cohort. Arthritis Rheumatol 68:1136–1144. https://doi.org/10.1002/art.39564
9. Veronese N, Stubbs B, Solmi M et al (2017) Association between lower limb osteoarthritis and incidence of depressive symptoms: data from the osteoarthritis initiative. Age Ageing 46:470. https://doi.org/10.1093/ageing/afw216
10. Veronese N, Stubbs B, Solmi M, Smith T et al (2018) Knee osteoarthritis and risk of hypertension: a longitudinal cohort study. Rejuvenation Res 21(1):15–21. https://doi.org/10.1089/rej.2017.1917
11. Veronese N, Stubbs B, Solmi M et al (2018) Osteoarthritis increases the risk of cardiovascular disease: data from the osteoarthritis initiative. J Nutr Health Aging 22:371. https://doi.org/10.1007/s12603-017-0941-0

12. Stubbs B, Aluko Y, Myint PK et al (2016) Prevalence of depressive symptoms and anxiety in osteoarthritis: a systematic review and meta-analysis. Age Ageing 45:228. https://doi.org/10.1093/ageing/afw001
13. Huang SW, Wang WT, Chou LC et al (2016) Osteoarthritis increases the risk of dementia: a nationwide cohort study in Taiwan. Sci Rep 5:10145. https://doi.org/10.1038/srep10145
14. Beaudart C, Biver E, Bruyere O et al (2018) Quality of life assessment in musculo-skeletal health. Aging Clin Exp Res 30(5):413–418. https://doi.org/10.1007/s40520-017-0794-8
15. Veronese N, Stubbs B, Noale M, Solmi M, Luchini C, Maggi S (2016) Adherence to the Mediterranean diet is associated with better quality of life: data from the osteoarthritis initiative. Am J Clin Nutr 104:1403–1409. https://doi.org/10.3945/ajcn.116.136390
16. Veronese N, Stubbs B, Noale M et al (2017) Adherence to a Mediterranean diet is associated with lower prevalence of osteoarthritis: data from the osteoarthritis initiative. Clin Nutr 36:1609. https://doi.org/10.1016/j.clnu.2016.09.035
17. Atukorala I, Makovey J, Lawler L et al (2016) Is there a dose-response relationship between weight loss and symptom improvement in persons with knee osteoarthritis? Arthritis Care Res 68:1106–1114
18. Bergink AP, Zillikens MC, Van Leeuwen JP et al (2016) 25-Hydroxyvitamin D and osteoarthritis: a meta-analysis including new data. Semin Arthritis Rheum 45:539–546. https://doi.org/10.1016/j.semarthrit.2015.09.010
19. Jin X, Jones G, Cicuttini F, Wluka A et al (2016) Effect of vitamin D supplementation on Tibial cartilage volume and knee pain among patients with symptomatic knee osteoarthritis: a randomized clinical trial. JAMA 315:1005–1013. https://doi.org/10.1001/jama.2016.1961
20. Trichopoulou A, Vasilopoulou E (2000) Mediterranean diet and longevity. Br J Nutr 84:S205–S209
21. Bartels EM, Juhl CB, Christensen R et al (2016) Aquatic exercise for the treatment of knee and hip osteoarthritis. Cochrane Database Syst Rev 3:CD005523. https://doi.org/10.1002/14651858.CD005523.pub3
22. Brosseau L, Taki J, Desjardins B, Thevenot O et al (2017) The Ottawa panel clinical practice guidelines for the management of knee osteoarthritis. Part three: aerobic exercise programs. Clin Rehabil 31:612–624. https://doi.org/10.1177/0269215517691085
23. Minshull C, Gleeson N (2017) Considerations of the principles of resistance training in exercise studies for the Management of Knee Osteoarthritis: a systematic review. Arch Phys Med Rehabil 98:1842. https://doi.org/10.1016/j.apmr.2017.02.026
24. Osteras N, Kjeken I, Smedslund G, Moe RH et al (2017) Exercise for hand osteoarthritis. Cochrane Database Syst Rev 1:CD010388. https://doi.org/10.1002/14651858.CD010388.pub2
25. Hui M, Doherty M, Zhang W (2011) Does smoking protect against osteoarthritis? Meta-analysis of observational studies. Ann Rheum Dis 70:1231–1237. https://doi.org/10.1136/ard.2010.142323
26. Dube CE, Liu SH, Driban JB, McAlindon TE et al (2016) The relationship between smoking and knee osteoarthritis in the osteoarthritis initiative. Osteoarthr Cartil 24:465–472. https://doi.org/10.1016/j.joca.2015.09.015
27. Cross M, Smith E, Hoy D et al (2015) The global burden of hip and knee osteoarthritis: estimates from the global burden of disease 2010 study. Ann Rheum Dis 73:1323–1330. https://doi.org/10.1136/annrheumdis-2013-204763

Postponing Cognitive Decline

13

Andreas U. Monsch, Panagiota Mistridis, and Alessandra Thomann

Key Messages

- Due to demographic change, dementia represents a major health care issue for our society.
- Although the underlying pathogenesis of AD is not fully understood, several observational studies provide strong evidence for an adverse effect of multiple cardiovascular and lifestyle risk factors.
- Prevention programs and strategies targeting the modification of these factors seem a viable and reasonable approach to mitigate and delay cognitive decline and dementia.
- Various factors including a healthy diet, smoking cessation, a physically active lifestyle and cognitive activity have been proposed to exert protective effects on both physical and mental health.
- The "Health Coaching" program developed by the Swiss College of Primary Care Medicine targeting multiple risk factors may in combination with "BrainCoach" represent a promising, long-term effective and low-cost approach to maintain both physical and mental health.

13.1 Introduction

The increase of life expectancy over the last century is paralleled by an elevated number of individuals with dementia, placing an enormous social and economic burden on society and health care systems, in addition to the devastating consequences for patients and their families. According to the World Alzheimer Report

A. U. Monsch (✉) · P. Mistridis · A. Thomann
Memory Clinic, University Center for Medicine of Aging Basel, Felix Platter Hospital, Basel, Switzerland
e-mail: Andreas.Monsch@unibas.ch

J.-P. Michel (ed.), *Prevention of Chronic Diseases and Age-Related Disability*, Practical Issues in Geriatrics, https://doi.org/10.1007/978-3-319-96529-1_13

2015, there is an estimated 47 million people worldwide suffering from dementia [1]. Based on current simulation models, the number of cases is expected to at least double every 20 years, reaching almost 132 million cases until 2050. However, recent reports suggest that the age-specific incidence of dementia might be decreasing in persons with at least high school diploma, possibly due to an improvement in cardiovascular health [2, 3]. Nevertheless and irrespective of how fast the growth of the number of people with dementia will be, the economic impact associated with dementia is huge and increasing. Worldwide, the current total costs have increased by 35% in the last 5 years and were estimated at US$ 818 billion in 2015, representing 1% of the global gross domestic product [1]. These costs include direct medical care costs (i.e., dementia treatment in primary and secondary care), direct social care costs (i.e., community care professionals and residential home setting), and informal care costs (i.e., unpaid care by family and others) [1].

Although several causes of dementia exist, we will focus this review on its most common cause, i.e., Alzheimer's disease (AD). Despite decades of research, the pathological mechanisms underlying this disease remain largely unclear. However, a broad consensus exists that AD has a complex multifactorial etiology and is modulated by various risk factors [4, 5]. A recent estimation calculated by Norton et al. [6] implies that, taking into account the interdependency of these factors, about one-third of AD cases worldwide may be attributable to seven potentially modifiable risk factors: diabetes, midlife hypertension, midlife obesity, depression, physical inactivity, smoking, and low educational attainment (see Fig. 13.1; see also [4]).

While current pharmacological and non-pharmacological treatments may decelerate disease progression, no curative or disease-modifying intervention exists to prevent the pathogenesis of dementia [7, 8]. Thus, there is a pressing need to identify preventive measures and strategies aiming to maintain brain health and delay cognitive decline. Importantly, as neurodegenerative disorders as AD have a long "silent" phase with no or only very subtle symptoms [9], such preventive programs should optimally be implemented at the earliest possible time when cognitive impairments are not yet manifested [10–12]. Figure 13.2 illustrates that preventive strategies require a lifespan perspective. Thus, children and adolescents need to be targeted with regard to education and, starting at midlife, optimal management of potential risk factors is essential [12].

Different modifiable factors to preserve cognitive health have been described. **A healthy diet** (e.g., Mediterranean) rich in antioxidants, vitamins (e.g., vitamin B12, E, and D), and polyunsaturated fatty acids (e.g., omega-3–[13]) may lower the risk of cognitive decline and dementia by reducing for example the risk for cardiovascular diseases. However, although findings from different studies suggest that specific dietary patterns or nutritional components may represent promising interventions in delaying cognitive decline, evidence in this regard is still weak and further investigation on this topic is needed [14, 15]. Additionally, also **physical activity** is known to exert beneficial effects on brain health. Promising results from different observational and intervention studies, as well as systematic reviews, examining the association between physical activity and the risk of cognitive impairment and dementia, yielded promising results with moderate to strong effects of physical activity on

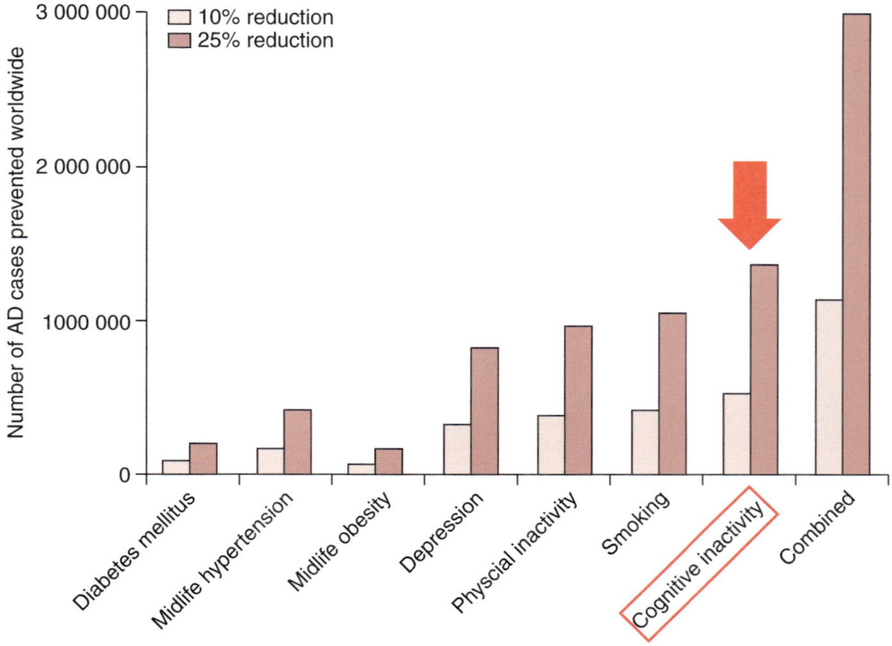

Fig. 13.1 Prevalence and estimates for population-attributable risks (PAR) for Alzheimer's disease (AD) in 2010 (Data source: Norton et al. [6]). PAR = population-attributable risk, i.e., the proportion of AD cases in the population that can be attributed to individual risk factors calculated by using the population prevalence and the relative risk of the risk factor. Combined = calculated prevalence and PAR for the seven individual risk factors combined, assuming independence of the risk factors. Adjusted combined = calculated prevalence and PAR for all seven risk factors combined with adjustment for non-independence of the risk factors

brain health. These results indicate that individuals with a physically active lifestyle exhibit less cognitive decline [16], reduced brain atrophy [17], and increased hippocampal volume [9] compared to people with a sedentary lifestyle. A third important protective factor for the maintenance of brain health is **cognitive activity**. This aspect will be reviewed in more detail below and a "BrainCoach" program, which focuses on cognitive activity as a preventive measure of cognitive decline, is introduced.

13.2 Cognitive Activity as a Modifiable Protective Factor for Cognitive Decline

As shown in Fig. 13.1, low educational attainment [6] or cognitive inactivity [4] constitutes the largest single risk factor for AD. Certainly, a high educational attainment will not prevent pathological brain changes. However, a number of studies indicate that higher educational attainment is related to higher levels of cognitive performance and seems to buffer negative effects and mitigate clinical symptoms in

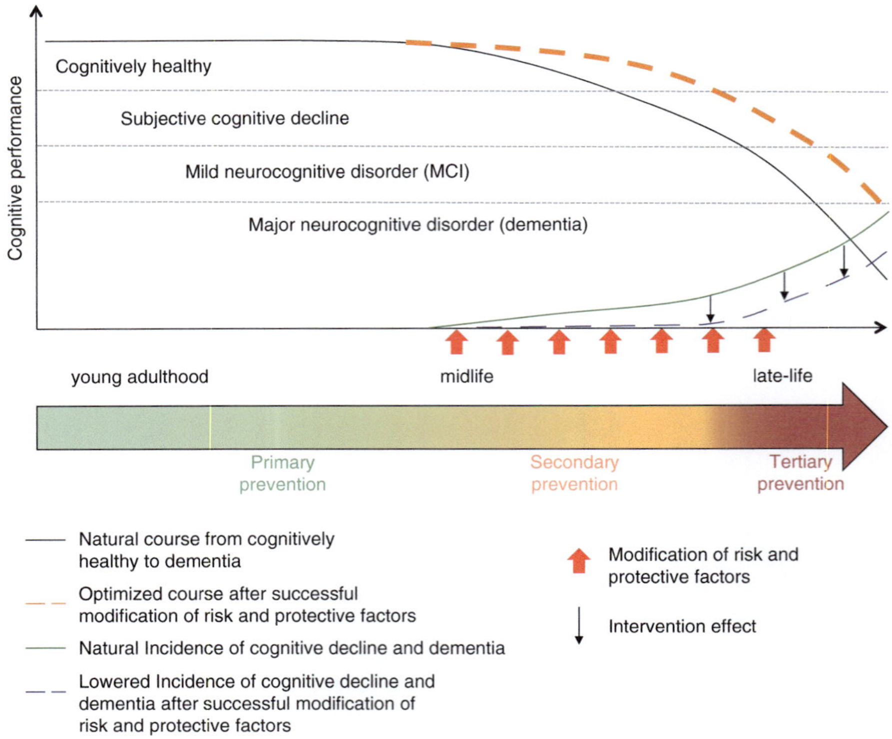

Fig. 13.2 Hypothesized model of neurocognitive disorders [12] across lifespan without (black line) and with (orange dashed line) successful modification of risk and protective factors and the consequence on dementia incidence rates: natural course (green line) vs. result of optimally timed preventive strategies through primary, secondary, and tertiary prevention (blue dashed line) (figure adapted from [36] (reproduced with permission), [18] (reproduced with permission: © 2014 The Association for the Publication of the Journal of Internal Medicine))

everyday life [2, 18, 19]. The rationale behind this observation is the hypothesis that higher educational attainment results in an increased cognitive reserve [18]. This so-called cognitive reserve hypothesis implies that individuals with higher levels of brain activity (e.g., through individual or synergistic contributions of high educational/occupational attainment and maintained cognitive activity up until old age) may better cope with brain pathology and are able to compensate brain damage much longer because of increased synaptic densities and a more complex and efficient structure of neural networks [18]. Thus, people with the same extent of pathological brain changes may exhibit different clinical manifestations of the disease depending on their level of cognitive reserve (see Fig. 13.3 [20]). Importantly, a person with a high cognitive reserve will have a steeper decline once symptoms are manifest due to higher pathological brain accumulations until cognitive dysfunctions are clinically perceivable [20].

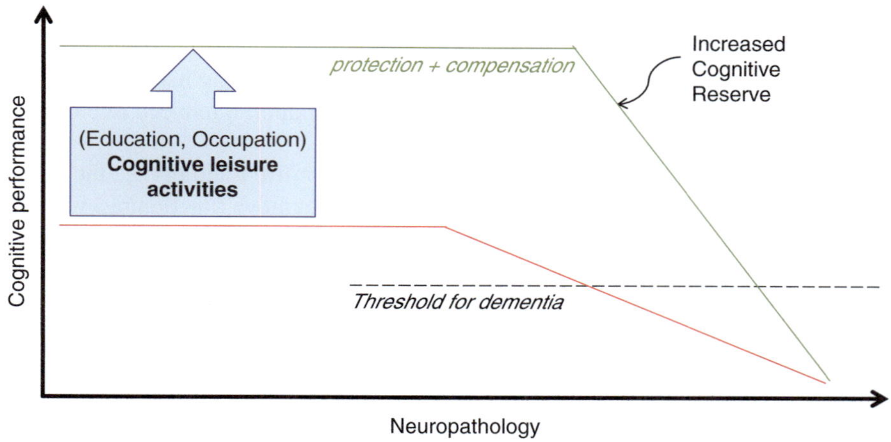

Fig. 13.3 Illustration of the association between the emergence of dementia-associated neuropathology, its clinical expression and cognitive reserve (figure adapted from [21]; reproduced with permission). Educational attainment and occupational challenges can usually no longer be changed in individuals aged 50 years and older. However, cognitive leisure activities may increase their cognitive reserve and thus lead to a delay in the emergence of cognitive decline

These findings are supported by several studies reporting reduced incidence rates of cognitive impairment and dementia in older adults with a high educational attainment [2, 19]. Additionally, an analysis from Barnes and Yaffe [4] indicates that the relative risk (i.e., the ratio of the probability to develop dementia in an at-risk group compared to a non-risk group) for dementia in people with a low education (i.e., with only primary education) is 59% higher compared to people with a higher education.

However, older adults experiencing a cognitive decline obviously already completed their formal and occupational education. The cognitive reserve, though, is not influenced by education alone. Retrospective studies indicate that significant associations exist between cognitively activating leisure activities, engagement in social activities, the level of cognitive performance, and the risk of dementia [21, 22]. Moreover, studies show that performing cognitively stimulating leisure activities later in life may somewhat compensate for a low educational attainment [23, 24]. Thus, cognitive reserve is not a static condition—it can be influenced and enhanced at any point in someone's lifetime.

There is great diversity of cognitive tasks and their duration of exposure in different studies investigating the association between cognitive activity and the risk of dementia. Thus, some studies also brought some inconclusive findings. Nevertheless, there is substantial evidence that participating in cognitive activities conveys beneficial effects for the maintenance of brain health and may delay cognitive decline [22]. Different experimental studies on rodents [25] and imaging studies on humans [26] suggest that a mentally stimulating environment promotes neurotrophic changes in the hippocampal formation, neurogenesis, and synaptic density. An imaging study by Valenzuela et al. [26] with healthy older human adults shows that participants with high levels of mental activities (in the domains of education, occupation, creative arts, reading, writing, socializing, and day-to-day habits) across the lifespan (young adulthood, middle age, and late life) exhibit a reduced rate of hippocampal atrophy compared to those with low levels.

A Cochrane review [27] examining the effect of cognitive training (i.e., the structured practice on tasks targeting specific domains of cognitive functioning) with 36 included studies involving healthy older participants or people with mild cognitive impairment provides evidence for an improvement in immediate and delayed verbal recall compared to participants without training. However, this positive effect did not exceed the improvements in active control groups receiving "only" unspecific cognitive stimulation such as reading, playing board games, or dancing that may significantly reduce the risk for cognitive decline or dementia (see also e.g., [28]). Moreover, various studies revealed that musical activities (i.e., playing an instrument or singing) enhance performance in different cognitive domains (attention, executive functions) by promoting neural plasticity and increasing gray matter volume in frontal, motor, parietal, and temporal (e.g., hippocampus) areas [29].

In summary, there is hopeful evidence that non-pharmacological interventions in stages with no or very little cognitive impairment may be effective in delaying (further) cognitive decline. Optimally, such a program should address all possible preventive aspects: dietary habits, physical activity, intake of toxic substances (smoking behavior and alcohol consumption), and cognitive activity.

13.3 Prevention Studies with a Multidimensional Approach

Although observational studies confirm the association between the mentioned modifiable risk factors and AD, results from intervention studies investigating the effect of these factors in delaying the onset of cognitive decline or AD are mixed. These inconsistent findings may have resulted from various methodological problems including small samples, short intervention periods with short follow-ups or inappropriate timing (too late to obtain a significant intervention effect; or a mono-interventional approach investigating only one risk factor [10]). However, as the underlying pathology of AD is multifactorial, measures addressing multiple target areas aiming to modify vascular and lifestyle factors simultaneously seem more appropriate. To date, there are three large ongoing European intervention studies targeting simultaneously multiple risk factors: the Finnish Geriatric Intervention Study to Prevent Cognitive Impairment and Disability (**FINGER**; [30, 31]), the Prevention of Dementia by Intensive Vascular Care (**PreDIVA**, [32]) study, and the study Multidomain Alzheimer Preventive Trial (**MAPT**, [33, 34]). Until now, only preliminary results from these studies have been published. In 2011, the European Dementia Prevention Initiative (**EDPI**; http://www.edpi.org/) was launched to combine the valuable information collected in the three ongoing European trials mentioned above. The aim of this initiative is to improve and promote the collaboration between researchers involved in the field of dementia prevention to combine experience and datasets and better define target populations, intervention strategies, and methodological challenges in large dementia prevention trials [10]. Based on the studies mentioned above, an innovative and interactive Internet intervention platform for the treatment of cardiovascular disease in older people was initiated as an additional project by the members of the EDPI called Healthy Aging Through Internet Counseling in the Elderly (**HATICE**; http://www.hatice.eu/). An additional initiative from Switzerland named **"EviPrev"** is based on current scientific data and focuses on evidence-based prevention and early detection of potentially chronic diseases (short interventions on physical activity, nutrition, smoking, alcohol consumption and screening for high blood pressure, dyslipidemia, diabetes, breast cancer, colon cancer, and others) in primary health care setting. Although this project is not considered to be a prevention study with a multidimensional approach, it has an important impact on cognitive health by systematically recording cardiovascular risk factors. A systematic assessment of these risk factors which significantly affect cognitive health is crucial for effective treatments and successful lifestyle interventions [35].

13.4 Health Coaching: A Multidimensional Counseling Program to Promote Health Behavior in the Primary Care Setting

Based on the findings summarized so far, an additional multidimensional and structured health program of counseling in primary care practice called "Health Coaching" was developed by the Swiss College of Primary Care Medicine (http://www.gesundheitscoaching-khm.ch/; [36]. Designed for GPs, the primary aim of this program is to promote health behavior in the Swiss population and prevent chronic diseases (e.g., stroke, coronary heart disease, cardiovascular disease) by targeting the most important contributors to disease burden including smoking, alcohol consumption, body weight, dietary habits, level of physical activity, and coping strategies with stress [36, 37]. The aim is to give GPs the tools to motivate their patients and accompany them during the implementation of a healthier lifestyle. Patients are involved in the decision process and share the responsibility for their health with the practitioner. Thus, an important aspect of "Health Coaching" is that patient and health professional meet on equal terms and jointly plan a step-by-step health program based on the patient's individual preferences and abilities [36]. The program also emphasizes the high importance of the GPs' communication skills and offers specific training programs in Motivational Interviewing (MI; see below) within this program [38]. Although Health Coaching as a non-pharmacological program is certainly quite comprehensive and probably sufficient for individuals who are still in work force, it could benefit from an additional module focusing on cognitive activity for patients who are beyond retirement or who exhibit subtle cognitive problems.

13.5 BrainCoach Program to Promote Cognitive Activity

13.5.1 Cognitive Activity

Based on scientific data reviewed above we have developed a cognitive activity program named "BrainCoach," which was specifically created for older adults at risk for cognitive impairment who might be e.g., in the so-called "silent phase" of AD [39] and is meant to be implemented in the primary care setting to be conducted by the GPs and other health care professionals (e.g., psychologists). The primary purpose of this module is—in accordance with the theory of cognitive reserve described above and the rule of "Use it or lose it!"—to accompany older adults and promote their motivation to maintain and increase brain health by increasing their cognitive activity. The program addresses especially older adults feeling cognitively "bored" in everyday life, individuals being shortly before retirement, or individuals with subtle cognitive alterations. The promotion of the activity will be achieved by a specific folder (A4-format) including information about cognitive activity and its effects on brain health, communication skills (Motivational Interviewing), and a structured questionnaire as a guideline (working sheet) to evaluate the patients' current cognitive activity and increase their motivation to find and implement a cognitive activity in their daily life. The "BrainCoach" program intentionally does not include specific cognitive exercises but highlights the importance of eliciting the patients' motivation to find a cognitive activity that they like to perform regularly (e.g., something they performed earlier in their life). In case the patients cannot think of any cognitive activity they would like to engage in, the "BrainCoach" program offers a range of different cognitive activities—a "cognitive buffet" (i.e., different activities depicted on color photographs)—from which the patients may choose the ones they would like to perform. Some possible activities can be performed individually such as doing artwork, solving crossword puzzles, singing, playing a musical instrument, or reading books/newspapers. Activities carried out in groups have an additional stimulating component, especially due to social interactions. Examples for these kinds of activities include language courses, dancing classes, singing in a choir, reading circles, attending university for seniors, playing board games, or attending cultural events with friends (e.g., theater, cinema, and concerts). This list included in the "BrainCoach" program cannot be complete, since a variety of additional activities may positively affect brain health. The patients are free in choosing something from this list or engage in another cognitively stimulating activity. The "BrainCoach" program is cost-free; however, the chosen activities have to be paid by the patients.

13.5.2 Motivational Interviewing (MI)

Mathematically speaking it would make the most sense to especially inspire patients with a low cognitive reserve to (newly) engage in cognitive activities, since these individuals have the largest room for improvement (see Fig. 13.3). Thus, the technique used to motivate patients will be critical. MI is a well-known client-centered and collaborative counseling technique that has frequently and successfully been applied in general health care settings and health promotion [40]. Briefly, eliciting people's intrinsic motivation appears to be a key factor to achieve long-lasting behavioral change [41–43]. For example, in the "BrainCoach" program a cognitive activity is chosen from the cognitive buffet because of the patient's personal interest in the activity. Its motivation is more likely to be intrinsic, because the patient probably chose this activity for being enjoyable, pleasurable, or giving satisfaction. Importantly, because patient and health practitioner work together at eye level to identify a suitable cognitive activity, engagement in this activity is not extrinsically motivated. That is, the patient does not engage in this activity to receive a reward, or because of feeling obliged. MI can be used in a brief intervention format, making it suitable for the primary care setting. As motivating and accompanying patients to make health-related behavioral changes represent a challenge for GPs, profound communication skills are crucial for successful counseling. Within the "BrainCoach" program, a training program for GPs in MI has been developed.

The "BrainCoach" program, including the folder, the "cognitive buffet," and a structured questionnaire (work sheet) based on the communication skills included in MI has been tested in a pilot study (feasibility, acceptance of the documents and the concept) and resulted in very high acceptance rates in both GPs and patients.

Conclusions

Due to demographic change, dementia represents a major health care issue for our society. Although the underlying pathogenesis of AD is not fully understood, a number of observational studies provide strong evidence for an adverse effect of multiple cardiovascular and lifestyle risk factors. In this regard, prevention strategies are needed to manage and lower the increase of dementia cases influenced by these risk factors. Delaying cognitive decline and dementia would have a huge impact on its incidence and prevalence. Specifically, a 10–20% reduction of the seven main risk factors for AD (diabetes, midlife hypertension, midlife obesity, physical inactivity, depression, smoking, low educational attainment) would decrease AD prevalence by 8–15% until 2050 [7]. Additionally, estimations from a projection model imply that interventions with the potential to delay disease onset or progression by only 1 year would reduce the number of AD patients by about 11% (i.e., nine million cases; [43]). Understanding the contribution and the impact of different lifestyle factors on disease development will have an important influence on future disease management and treatment since many of these risk factors are modifiable.

Disclosure The "BrainCoach" program is financially supported by an unrestricted grant from Vifor Pharma, Switzerland.

References

1. Alzheimer's Disease International (2015) World Alzheimer Report 2015. The global impact of dementia. [Internet]. Available from: http://www.alz.co.uk/research/WorldAlzheimerReport2015.pdf
2. Satizabal CL, Beiser AS, Chouraki V et al (2016) Incidence of dementia over three decades in the Framingham Heart Study. N Engl J Med 374:523–532
3. Matthews FE, Stephan BCM, Robinson L et al (2016) A two decade dementia incidence comparison from the cognitive function and ageing studies I and II. Nat Commun 7:11398
4. Barnes DE, Yaffe K (2011) The projected effect of risk factor reduction on Alzheimer's disease prevalence. Lancet Neurol 10:819–828
5. Xu W, Tan L, Wang H-F, Jiang T, Tan M-S, Tan L et al (2015) Meta-analysis of modifiable risk factors for Alzheimer's disease. J Neurol Neurosurg Psychiatry 86(12):1299–1306
6. Norton S, Matthews FE, Barnes DE et al (2014) Potential for primary prevention of Alzheimer's disease: an analysis of population-based data. Lancet Neurol 13:788–794
7. Andrieu S, Coley N, Lovestone S et al (2015) Prevention of sporadic Alzheimer's disease: lessons learned from clinical trials and future directions. Lancet Neurol 14:926–944
8. Barnett J, Bahar-Fuchs A, Cherbuin N, Herath P, Anstey K (2015) Interventions to prevent cognitive decline and dementia in adults without cognitive impairment: a systematic review. J Prev Alzheimers Dis 2:38–44
9. Erickson KI, Voss MW, Prakash RS et al (2011) Exercise training increases size of hippocampus and improves memory. Proc Natl Acad Sci 108:3017–3022
10. Richard E, Andrieu S, Solomon A et al (2012) Methodological challenges in designing dementia prevention trials—the European dementia prevention initiative (EDPI). J Neurol Sci 322:64–70
11. Solomon A, Mangialasche F, Richard E et al (2014) Advances in the prevention of Alzheimer's disease and dementia. J Intern Med 275:229–250
12. Biessels GJ (2014) Capitalising on modifiable risk factors for Alzheimer's disease. Lancet Neurol 13:752–753
13. Morris MC, Tangney CC, Wang Y et al (2015) MIND diet associated with reduced incidence of Alzheimer's disease. Alzheimers Dement 11:1007–1014
14. Gillette-Guyonnet S, Secher M, Vellas B (2013) Nutrition and neurodegeneration: epidemiological evidence and challenges for future research. Br J Clin Pharmacol 75:738–755
15. Canevelli M, Lucchini F, Quarata F et al (2016) Nutrition and dementia: evidence for preventive approaches? Nutrients 8:144
16. Hayes SM, Alosco ML, Hayes JP et al (2015) Physical activity is positively associated with episodic memory in aging. J Int Neuropsychol Soc 21:780–790
17. Best JR, Chiu BK, Liang Hsu C et al (2015) Long-term effects of resistance exercise training on cognition and brain volume in older women: results from a randomized controlled trial. J Int Neuropsychol Soc 21.(Special Issue 10:745–756
18. Stern Y (2012) Cognitive reserve in ageing and Alzheimer's disease. Lancet Neurol 11:1006–1012
19. Langa C, Larson EB, Crimmins E et al (2017) A comparison of the prevalence of dementia in the United States in 2000 and 2012. JAMA Intern Med 177:51–58
20. Stern Y (2009) Cognitive reserve. Neuropsychologia 47:2015–2028
21. Sattler C, Toro P, Schönknecht P, Schröder J (2012) Cognitive activity, education and socioeconomic status as preventive factors for mild cognitive impairment and Alzheimer's disease. Psychiatry Res 196:90–95
22. Akbaraly TN, Portet F, Fustinoni S et al (2009) Leisure activities and the risk of dementia in the elderly: results from the Three-City Study. Neurology 73:854–861
23. Lachman ME, Agrigoroaei S, Murphy C et al (2010) Frequent cognitive activity compensates for education differences in episodic memory. Am J Geriatr Psychiatry 18:4–10

24. Reed BR, Dowling M, Tomaszewski Farias S et al (2011) Cognitive activities during adulthood are more important than education in building reserve. J Int Neuropsychol Soc 17:615–624
25. Woods B, Aguirre E, Spector AE et al (2012) Cognitive stimulation to improve cognitive functioning in people with dementia. Cochrane Database Syst Rev (2):CD005562
26. Valenzuela MJ, Sachdev P, Wen W et al (2008) Lifespan mental activity predicts diminished rate of hippocampal atrophy. PLoS One 3:e2598
27. Martin M, Clare L, Altgassen AM et al (2011) Cognition-based interventions for healthy older people and people with mild cognitive impairment. Cochrane Database Syst Rev 1:CD006220
28. Stern C, Munn Z (2010) Cognitive leisure activities and their role in preventing dementia: a systematic review. Int J Evid Based Healthc 8:2–17
29. Fotuhi M, Do D, Jack C (2012) Modifiable factors that alter the size of the hippocampus with ageing. Nat Rev Neurol 8:189–202
30. Kivipelto M, Ngandu T, Laatikainen T et al (2006) Risk score for the prediction of dementia risk in 20 years among middle aged people: a longitudinal, population-based study. Lancet Neurol 5:735–741
31. Ngandu T, Lehtisalo J, Solomon A et al (2015) A 2 year multidomain intervention of diet, exercise, cognitive training, and vascular risk monitoring versus control to prevent cognitive decline in at-risk elderly people (FINGER): a randomised controlled trial. Lancet 385:2255–2263
32. Ligthart SA, van den Eerenbeemt KD, Pols J et al (2015) Perspectives of older people engaging in nurse-led cardiovascular prevention programmes: a qualitative study in primary care in the Netherlands. Br J Gen Pract 65:e41–e48
33. Lilamand M, Cesari M, Del Campo N et al (2016) Brain amyloid deposition is associated with lower instrumental activities of daily living abilities in older adults. Results from the MAPT study. J Gerontol A Biol Sci Med Sci 71:391–397
34. Vellas B, Carrie I, Gillette-Guyonnet S et al (2014) MAPT study: a multidomain approach for preventing Alzheimer's disease: design and baseline data. J Prev Alzheimers Dis 1:13–22
35. Cornuz J, Auer R, Neuner-Jehle S et al (2015) Schweizer Empfehlungen für den Check-up in der Arztpraxis. Swiss Med Forum 15:974–980
36. Neuner-Jehle S, Schmid M, Grüninger U (2013) The "Health Coaching" programme: a new patient-centred and visually supported approach for health behaviour change in primary care. BMC Fam Pract 14:1–8
37. Neuner-Jehle S, Schmid M, Grüninger U (2014) Kurzberatung in der Arztpraxis zur Verbesserung des Gesundheitsverhaltens: probleme und Lösungen. Praxis 103:271–277
38. Neuner-Jehle S, Grüninger U, Schmid M (2016) Efficacy of a communication skill training fostering health promotion in primary care: a mixed method analysis. 2161–0711
39. Dubois B, Hampel H, Feldman HH et al (2016) Preclinical Alzheimer's disease: definition, natural history, and diagnostic criteria. Alzheimers Dement 12:292–323
40. Söderlund LL, Madson MB, Rubak S et al (2011) A systematic review of motivational interviewing training for general health care practitioners. Patient Educ Couns 84:16–26
41. Ng JYY, Ntoumanis N, Thøgersen-Ntoumani C et al (2012) Self-determination theory applied to health contexts a meta-analysis. Perspect Psychol Sci 7:325–340
42. Patrick H, Resnicow K, Teixeira PJ et al (2013) Chapter 5—communication skills to elicit physical activity behavior change: how to talk to the client. ACSMs Health Fit J:129–149
43. Teixeira PJ, Silva MN, Mata J et al (2012) Motivation, self-determination, and long-term weight control. Int J Behav Nutr Phys Act 9:22

14 Age-Related Decline of Vision, Hearing, and Balance: Pathophysiology and Midlife Prevention

Patrice Tran Ba Huy

Key Messages

- Starting around the fourth decade, structural changes affect the retina and peripheral nerve fibers, susceptible to provoke later dysfunctions in daily life.
- Midlife examination could detect eye diseases, acquired or genetic with late revelation, liable to exacerbate the adverse effects of aging. At this age, controlling also external risk factors is very important.
- Starting between 40 and 50 years, age-related hearing loss (presbycusis) has a high prevalence, doubling with each successive age decade and affecting over two-thirds of adults aged over 70 years.
- As there is no treatment for presbycusis, midlife prevention is essential and mainly based on the management of the extrinsic factors: mainly drug-induced ototoxicity and chronic acoustic trauma.
- Balance degenerative changes, linked to alterations of peripheral sensory systems (vestibular, visual, and proprioceptive), central structures integrating sensory input and motor systems (skeletal/oculomotor/somatic muscles), affect more than a quarter the 65+ population and about half of those 85+.
- Prevention of balance disorder is of utmost importance. It is founded on midlife examination screening for risk factors and comorbidities, correcting any environmental and lifestyle problems and, above all, recommending physical activity.

Vision, hearing, and balance play major roles in our daily life. With age, these sensory systems tend to lose function, not only because of the biology of aging but also through independent mechanisms unique to each of them [1]. In other words, sensory decline is an inevitable physiological process which is aggravated by some

P. Tran Ba Huy
French National Academy of Medicine, Paris, France
e-mail: patrice.tran-ba-huy@aphp.fr

J.-P. Michel (ed.), *Prevention of Chronic Diseases and Age-Related Disability*, Practical Issues in Geriatrics, https://doi.org/10.1007/978-3-319-96529-1_14

specific etiologic factors. Prevention is essential to minimize major geriatric outcomes including physical, cognitive, and socioeconomic aspects.

In this chapter, we discuss the respective pathophysiology of the decline of these sensory functions and the measures aiming at preventing, or more precisely delaying, the impact of age and at promoting healthy aging and quality of life.

14.1 Vision

Starting around the fourth decade, structural changes affect the retina and peripheral nerve fibers: loss of cones and rods, reduction of pupil diameter, senile miosis, slowing of the pupillary reflex, yellowing of the crystalline lens, etc. [2]. These alterations impair several system functions, including field of view, acuity, color discrimination, contrast sensitivity at high spatial frequencies, depth and motion perception, visual processing speed, etc.

As a result, visual dysfunction has a significant impact on daily living, including mobility-based activities and quality of life. A large body of evidence suggests that diminished visual information, whatever its cause, is associated with increased risk of falls [3] and may affect vision-dependent cognitive outcomes. Some studies [4, 5] suggested that individuals with advanced age-related macular degeneration (AMD) have a greater 2-year risk of developing Alzheimer's disease than those with better vision. Conversely, deficits in visual cognition in Alzheimer patients have been widely reported. Finally, some studies have shown that visual stimulus enhancement has a positive impact on many aspects of the functional impairments experienced by patients with Alzheimer's disease [6].

Clinically, impaired accommodation is the most sensitive and earliest index of age-related vision impairment. Unfortunately this physiological process, known as presbyopia, too often leads to self-correction by over-the-counter "reading glasses," without medical prescription. Apart from the problems of optical error and poor centering, especially frequent with progressive lenses, this bad habit, which is increasingly widespread and encouraged by mass retailers and the Internet, deprives the patient of a proper ophthalmologic assessment. Midlife examination could detect eye diseases, acquired or genetic with late revelation, liable to exacerbate the adverse effects of aging. There are two such pathologies which have particularly significant impact.

Measurement of ocular pressure could disclose chronic glaucoma, which, by contrast with acute glaucoma, may be revealed only by slow progressive deterioration of the visual field, with no reddish eye, pain, or loss of visual acuity. Fundus examination can diagnose retinopathy, which is a severe side-effect of diabetes and develops in nearly all individuals who have type I diabetes with more than 15 years' progression and in 50–80% of type II diabetic patients after 20 years [7].

Cataract and AMD are two major causes of vision loss, developing in older adults. However, the fact that they could have some genetic origin may justify genetic consultation for at-risk families.

Alongside these specific ophthalmologic pathologies, there are also general and environmental risk factors: (1) high blood pressure, diabetes, too-rich diet, sedentary lifestyle, and/or obesity increase the risk of eye-stroke; (2) prolonged excessive use of psychotropic drugs and/or antidepressants is the leading cause of dry eye in France; (3) alcohol abuse and smoking are known to induce optic neuropathy; (4) ultraviolet radiation exposure leads to phototoxicity more often than to phototrauma [8].

To summarize, midlife prevention of age-related decline of vision relies on systematic ophthalmologic evaluation and general measures in individuals over 45 years of age. Independently of specific treatment of any given ocular pathology and correction of extrinsic factors, non-pharmacological approaches such as enhancing the contrast and strength of visual stimuli could alleviate functional impairment in daily activities and, in the long term, postpone cognitive decline.

14.2 Hearing

Age-related hearing loss, known as presbycusis, has high prevalence, doubling with each successive age decade, with onset beginning around the 40s or 50s and affecting over two-thirds of adults aged over 70 years. According to epidemiological studies, it is the third most prevalent chronic medical affection after osteoarthritis and hypertension and has major, although underestimated, social and medical implications as it increases the risk of physical and cognitive (Lin) decline.

As in other sensory systems, presbycusis involves both intrinsic and extrinsic factors [4, 9].

Intrinsic factors include genetic and structural components. (1) Three genes, *KCNQ4* (encoding a voltage-gated potassium channel), *NAT2* (N-acetyl-transferase), and *GRM7* (glutamate metabotropic receptor 7), are considered susceptibility genes for presbycusis. This could account for the differences in susceptibility among older individuals, some presenting remarkable auditory performance with good speech discrimination whereas others develop early hearing impairment. (2) Inner and outer hair cells are limited in number and highly differentiated. These post-mitotic cells are unable to multiply; accordingly any loss, whatever its cause, is irreversible, leaving "dead zones" in the organ of Corti.

Extrinsic factors comprise two main etiologies. (1) Drug-induced ototoxicity mainly implicates aminoglycosides [10]. Their action mechanism is not fully elucidated, but at least partly involves individual genetic susceptibility. (2) Chronic acoustic trauma has been pinpointed since the seminal report by Rosen et al. In the 1960s, they found that 80–90-year-olds in a tribal community in Sudan showed hearing performances comparable to those of teenagers in New York; their tribal culture featured a low-fat low-protein diet and a quiet environment, their music involving no percussion instruments [11]. This surprising observation suggested that the noise of modern city life jeopardizes hearing.

Medical factors, such as diabetes, atherosclerosis, and viral infection, may have exacerbating effects. Whatever the factors involved, the final result is intracellular accumulation of free radicals, leading to apoptosis.

Histopathological studies identified four types of presbycusis, each presenting specific audiometric and etiologic features [12]. (1) The most frequent is *metabolic,* involving the stria vascularis. This microangiopathy affects the structure underlying the electrochemical characteristics of the endolymph bathing the organ of Corti. The audiometric curve is flat or slightly descending, with good speech discrimination. (2) The *neuronal type* involves the afferent fibers and spiral ganglion. The audiometric curve is descending, affecting high frequencies. (3) The *sensory type* predominantly affects hair cells, and especially the outer hair cells, leading to loss of frequency selectivity. The audiometric curve shows an abrupt drop at high frequencies. Experimental data suggest that this type is mainly caused by environmental noise. (4) The *mechanical type* results from age-related rigidity of the basilar membrane supporting the organ of Corti. The consequences are notably experienced by musicians, who begin tuning their instruments to ever-higher frequencies.

Clinically, the most common and earliest complaint in age-related hearing loss is difficulty in understanding speech, especially in the presence of background noise (the "cocktail party" effect). This symptom is due to poor frequency resolution of sounds by an impaired cochlea, and to higher-level cognitive factors. Impaired communication leads to socio-familial isolation, withdrawal, depression, etc. A major issue in this regard is that hearing loss in older adults may incur a long-term risk of dementia [13–15], with a shared neuropathologic etiology including synaptic alterations in central pathways, deficits in central auditory processing which in turn affect executive functions, and auditory difficulties requiring greater cognitive resources to process auditory perception, to the detriment of other cognitive processes such as working memory. Conversely, recent studies have suggested that patients with normal cognitive function carrying the APOEε4 allele, the most robust genetic risk allele for Alzheimer's disease, show significantly more severe presbycusis than non-carriers [4]. A convincing argument for a relationship between presbycusis and dementia was provided by a recent study suggesting that early rehabilitation by hearing aids postpones onset of the dementia; this finding awaits replication [16, 17].

Midlife prevention is mainly based on the management of the above extrinsic factors. Indications for aminoglycoside antibiotics are now well defined and limited. However, many other drugs are potentially ototoxic. Therefore, careful review of dosage, drug interactions, and the necessity of prescription are mandatory to limit auditory side-effects. Regarding acoustic trauma, it is well established that certain occupations, such as roadworkers and disk jockeys, and certain leisure activities, such as hunting, clay-pigeon shooting, and concert-going, should be the subject of strict and perhaps legally mandatory acoustic protection; it is impossible to overstate the dangers of the prolonged daily acoustic exposure suffered (and/or actively sought) by teenagers addicted to their headphones and earphones and the need for precise information on the risks involved.

Limiting the deleterious impact of these extrinsic factors is essential, especially since there is no curative treatment for presbycusis [18]. At the present time, hearing aids are the only means of palliating the decline of auditory function. However, there are many barriers to this solution: high cost, inadequate national health and private insurance cover, the inconvenience of repeated consultation for fitting and adjustments, and, above all, psychological unwillingness to accept reality. From a public health perspective, efforts should be made to increase the affordability and accessibility of sound amplifiers. For those who cannot benefit from amplification devices due to socioeconomic reasons, cognitive impairment, or problems of manual dexterity, other listening aids may be of great help: devices providing warnings and signals, headphones, amplified telephones, etc. Finally, education and coaching on the use of communication strategies must be undertaken: e.g., speaking face-to-face, reducing background noise, speaking more slowly.

To summarize, midlife prevention of age-related hearing decline is founded on careful protection of a limited auditory cell stock that is sadly sensitive to environmental aggression.

14.3 Balance

Balance disorder is becoming a major issue in developed countries [4, 19, 20], firstly because prevalence increases steadily with age, affecting a quarter to one-third of the population older than 65 years and about half of those older than 85. Secondly, over and above the everyday nuisance, it is a major risk factor for iterative falls, the devastating physical and financial consequences of which are notorious: 30% of adults older than 65 years fall at least once a year, and about 50% fall again, leading to hospital admission, restricted mobility, loss of independence, and a financial burden averaging $20 billion per year in the USA.

Pathophysiologically, balance in humans involves a complex system, including three peripheral sensory systems (vestibular, visual, and proprioceptive), and central structures integrating peripheral sensory input and transmitting appropriate commands to a select group of skeletal, oculomotor, and somatic muscles. The outcome of this system should be an automatic, unconscious, and instantaneous corporal response to spatial modifications accompanying movement: i.e., to stabilize posture and gaze.

With age, the whole balance system undergoes degenerative changes [21]. In the vestibule, loss of hair cells, disintegration of otoconia, decrease in the number of primary vestibular neurons, and shrinkage of vestibular nuclei have been extensively documented and attributed partly to microvascular changes. These structural alterations are confirmed by vestibular tests showing diminished vestibulo-ocular reflex, deterioration of the velocity storage mechanism, and delay in otolithic response. Concomitantly, the decline of visual performance affects the visual preponderance, which increases with age, older adults increasingly relying on the visual system to stabilize their posture. Similarly, aging of the muscles, joints, and tendons impairs proprioceptive system performance, as demonstrated by decreased stability on posturographic test and lowering of vibration and touch thresholds. In addition, reduction in strength and contraction speed, along with fatigability of skeletal, somatic and oculomotor muscles, delays the reaction to postural disturbance, as demonstrated by dynamic posturography and impaired saccadic, optokinetic and pursuit eye movements.

Concomitantly, the central structures (cerebellum, brainstem, and cortical structures) which integrate and stratify all these peripheral sensory inputs show progressive and irreversible changes, including demyelination, neuronal degeneration, etc.

Clinically, age-related dizziness (also known as presbystasis) induces a variety of symptoms and signs. Firstly, difficulty walking, slower gait speed, and shorter step length are universally reported by older individuals subject to dizziness. Secondly, constant fear of falling, anxiety, feeling unsafe, and lightheadedness constitute a heavy emotional burden that comes with vestibular loss, restricting daily activities and causing social isolation [20]. And thirdly, emerging literature suggests that difficulties in concentration and memory, leading to cognitive impairment, are associated with loss of balance.

Prevention of balance disorder and of its dramatic consequence, falls, includes analysis of the patient's environment and lifestyle, and thorough multidisciplinary screening for risk factors that worsen the deleterious side-effects of aging and should be identified and corrected as early as possible [22].

Environmental factors that may contribute to disorientation and increase the risk of falling should be identified: irregular flooring at home (rugs and carpets, steps, paving), insufficient lighting, unsuitable footwear (high heels, foam soles absorbing proprioceptive sensation, etc.), familial and social isolation, etc.

Physical examination should investigate the various systems involved in the maintenance of balance. Peripheral vestibular disorders including benign peripheral paroxysmal vertigo, Ménière's disease, vestibular neuritis, ototoxic insult, or any type of otologic pathology may aggravate or decompensate a precarious and aging balance system. Caloric and posturographic tests are baseline examinations.

Ophthalmologic check-up includes visual field and acuity, fundus examination and oculomotor function. It screens for incipient peripheral visual disorder (vascular optical neuropathy, glaucoma, or diabetic retinopathy), which disturbs balance more than central visual disorders such as AMD or cataract. Likewise, oculomotor disorder, as found in Parkinson's disease, impairs the visual scanning of surroundings that is so essential to balance. It is also worth stressing the dangers of progressive lenses, which heighten disorientation and the risk of falling.

The main neurologic pathologies leading to risk of fall are neurodegenerative diseases such as Parkinson's or Alzheimer's, normal pressure hydrocephaly, pseudobulbar conditions, and cerebellar syndrome. Higher mental function should also be assessed on questionnaires, particularly exploring memory deficit and cognitive decline and screening for psychogenic factors such as depression or fear of falling in itself, which is a vicious circle that progressively confines the elderly subject to immobility, only worsening the situation.

Orthopedic examination assesses muscle strength and osteoarticular freedom and flexibility, and screens for vertebral stasis disorder, flexion contracture of the hip, plantar abnormality and, more generally, history of trauma, and any disorder impairing proprioception or automatic compensatory muscle action accounting for maladapted motor response.

Finally, general evaluation should assess the patient's physical faculties and ability to perform the actions of everyday living. Two simple maneuvers should be implemented in any individual above 45 years of age: the Get-up-and-Go test (subject, seated on a chair with a back 3 m from a wall, gets up and heads for the wall to touch it, turns round, comes back to and circles the chair, then sits down again, all within 20 s or so), and the unipodal test (patient should stay upright for at least 5 s on a single leg).

Cardiovascular diathesis, osteoporosis, atherosclerosis, diabetes, recent anesthesia or confinement to bed, for however short a time, should be screened because such episodes are often followed by decompensation of central origin, from which elderly subjects cannot recover.

But it must also, and above all, be ensured that any medication, whatever the intercurrent pathologies, should not be excessive: the effects of sedatives, antidepressants, hypnotics, diuretics, and antihypertensives can cumulate and directly impair residual physical capacity; such iatrogenic effects are too often overlooked yet all too frequent.

To summarize, prevention of balance disorder is of utmost importance. It is founded on midlife examination screening for risk factors and comorbidities, correcting any environmental and lifestyle problems and, above all, recommending physical activity.

References

1. Gadkaree SK, Sun DQ, Li C et al (2016) Does sensory function decline independently or concomitantly with age? Data from the Baltimore longitudinal study of aging. J Aging Res 2016:1865038
2. Owsley C (2016) Vision and aging. Annu Rev Vis Sci 2:255–271
3. Crews JE, Chou CF, Sekar S et al (2017) The prevalence of chronic conditions and poor health among people with and without vision impairment, aged>65 years. Am J Ophthalmol 182:18–30
4. Albers MW, Gilmore GC, Kaye J et al (2015) At the interface of sensory and motor dysfunctions and Alzheimer's disease. Alzheimers Dement 11:70–98
5. Clemons TE, Rankin MW, McBee WL (2006) Cognitive impairment in the age-related disease study. Arch Ophtalmol 124:537–543
6. Cronin-Golomb A, Gilmore GC, Neargarder S et al (2007) Enhanced stimulus strength improves visual cognition in aging and Alzheimer's disease. Cortex 43:952–966
7. Klein R, Klein BE, Moss SE et al (1984) Prevalence and risk of diabetic retinopathy when age at diagnosis is less than 30 years. Arch Ophtalmol 102:520–526
8. Arné JL, Duffier JL, Hamard H et al (2013) La prise en charge des soins ophtalmologiques en France. Bull Acad Natl Med 137:1051–1053
9. Gates GA, Mills JH (2005) Presbycusis. Lancet 366:1111–1120
10. Hawkins JE (1973) Comparative pathology. Aging, noise and ototoxic drugs. Adv Otorhinolaryngol 20:125–141
11. Rosen G (1974) A backward glance at noise pollution. Am J Public Health 64:514–517
12. Schuknecht HF (1974) Pathology of the ear. Harvard University Press, Cambridge, MA
13. Gates GA, Beiser A, Rees TS et al (2002) Central auditory dysfunction may precede the onset of clinical dementia in people with probable Alzheimer's disease. J Am Geriatr Soc 50:482–488
14. Dartigues JF, Féart C (2011) Risk factors for Alzheimer disease: aging beyond age? Neurology 77:206–207

15. Lin FR, Yaffe K, Xia J et al (2013) Hearing loss and cognitive decline in older adults. JAMA Intern Med 173:293–299
16. Amieva H, Ouvrard C, Giulioli C et al (2015) Self-reported hearing loss, hearing aids, and cognitive decline in elderly adults: a 25-year study. J Am Geriatr Soc 63:2099–2104
17. "Dementia prevention, intervention, and care". http://www.thelancet.com/commissions/dementia2017
18. Mamo SK, Reed NS, Nieman CL et al (2016) Personal sound amplifiers for adults. Am J Med 129:245–250
19. Barin K, Dodson EE (2011) Dizziness in the elderly. Otolaryngol Clin N Am 44:437–454
20. Harun A, Semenov Y, Agrawal Y (2015) Vestibular function and activities of daily living. Gerontol Geriatr Med 1:2333721415607124
21. Rosenhall U, Rubin W (1975) Degenerative changes in the human vestibular sensory epithelia. Acta Otolaryngol 79:67–80
22. Tran Ba Huy P (2011) Troubles de l'équilibre du sujet âgé. Rev Prat 61:819–822

Fall Prevention

15

Hubert Blain, Pierre Louis Bernard, Chokri Boubakri, and Jean Bousquet

Key Messages

- 30% of people aged over 65 years fall each year; falls are one of the leading causes for hospitalization, disability, and admission to a nursing home.
- People who fall, or report recurrent falls in the past year, or demonstrate abnormalities of gait and/or balance should be considered at high risk of falling to be offered a multifactorial falls risk assessment.
- Individualized, targeted multifactorial interventions comprise the management of specific causes of gait/balance and muscle strength disturbances, prescription of vitamin D supplements, measures to improve home safety, a review of medications, vision optimization, insertion of a pacemaker in case of carotid sinus hypersensitivity, and multifaceted podiatry.
- Group and home-based exercise programmes that combine balance and moderate intensity strength training are effective to reduce falls in older people whatever the risk of falling.
- Design modifications to public environment including "age-friendly" transportation modifications and measures to enhance "fall awareness" in older people and health-care professionals are also necessary to prevent falls and their complications.

H. Blain (✉)
Department of Internal Medicine and Geriatrics, University Hospital of Montpellier, Montpellier University, Montpellier, France

MACVIA France, EA 2991, Euromov, Montpellier University, Montpellier, France

Centre de Prévention et de Traitement des Maladies du Vieillissement Antonin Balmès, Centre Hospitalier Universitaire de Montpellier, Montpellier, France
e-mail: h-blain@chu-montpellier.fr

P. L. Bernard · C. Boubakri · J. Bousquet
Department of Internal Medicine and Geriatrics, University Hospital of Montpellier, Montpellier University, Montpellier, France

MACVIA France, EA 2991, Euromov, Montpellier University, Montpellier, France

J.-P. Michel (ed.), *Prevention of Chronic Diseases and Age-Related Disability*, Practical Issues in Geriatrics, https://doi.org/10.1007/978-3-319-96529-1_15

15.1 Epidemiology of Falls

Among people living in the community approximately 30% of those aged over 65 years of age and 50% of those older than 80 fall each year and one-third of them are repeated fallers. Approximately 30% of falls result in an injury that requires medical attention, including fractures in approximately 10% and hip fractures in 2% of falls. Approximately 2.3 million of European citizens aged 65+ attend emergency departments each year with fall-related injuries (3% of all Europeans aged 65+), 1.5 million are admitted to hospital for fall-related injuries (it represents 60% of all causes of injury emergency ward attendance), and 36.000 die from falls. Falls are one of the leading causes for hospitalization and the third leading cause of disability. Falls can also have psychological consequences, including fear of falling and loss of confidence resulting in self-restricted activity levels, reduction in physical function and social interactions. Falling puts also a strain on the family and is an independent predictor of admission to a nursing home [1].

The fall rate in nursing homes is much higher than in ambulatory older subjects (respectively 2 and 1.5 falls per person-year in men and women,) with almost half of residents falling more than once a year [2, 3]. In nursing homes, the mean admission rate reaches 1 per person-year and fall-related admissions count for 15% of overall admissions. Confirmed diagnoses of fractures of the femur account for 10% of overall admissions and fracture incidence is between 1 and 4% in nursing homes [3].

Falls account also for up to 70% of inpatient accidents. Approximately 30% of hospital patient's falls result in physical injury, with 4–6% resulting in serious injury [4].

15.2 Cost of Falls in Subjects Aged 65 or Older

In the European Union, healthcare expenditures for treating fall-related injuries is estimated to be € 25 billion each year. Furthermore, shifting demographics over the next 35 years could result in annual fall-related expenditures exceeding € 45 billion by the year 2050 [1].

Fractures lead to 80% of the fall-related healthcare costs. The mean costs per fall are € 10,000, higher for women than men and increase with age. Persons aged 80+ account for almost 50% of all fall-related emergency department visits, and 66% of total costs [5].

The costs of long-term care at home and in nursing homes show the largest age-related increases and accounts together for 54% of the fall-related costs in older people [6].

15.3 How to Identify Subjects at Risk of Fall

15.3.1 Risk Factors of Falls

Risk factors of falls in community-dwelling older subjects include a fall history in the previous year, a fear of falling, a feeling of unsteadiness when walking, and intrinsic (such as age, female gender, leg weakness, and gait/balance disorders, incontinence, sadness or depression, vision disturbances, and cognitive impairment, especially) and extrinsic factors (such as environmental hazards, medications including psychotropic drugs). The American STEADI group recommends that people aged 65+ should fill in a questionnaire based on those risk factors, named *Stay independent brochure*, including questions on their history of fall in the previous year, balance/walking disturbances (need of a cane or a walker to get around safely, feeling of unsteadiness when walking, need to hold onto furniture when walking at home, fear of falling), muscle weakness (need to push with the hands to stand up from a chair, troubles stepping up onto a curb), urinary problems (need to rush to the toilets), numbness in the feet (some feeling loss in the feet), medications at risk of falling (use of drugs that make feel light-headed, more tired than usual, sleepy or antidepressant drugs), signs of depression or sadness (https://www.cdc.gov/steadi/pdf/stay_independent_brochure-a.pdf).

Subjects with a history of fall in the previous year, who feel unsteady when standing or walking, and subjects who scored 4/12 points or more should be considered at risk of falling and should get a strength/gait/balance assessment [7].

15.3.2 Tests to Assess Gait and Balance

According to the American and British Geriatrics Societies, tests of balance and gait may use the Timed up and go test (TUG) and the "turn 180°" test (TT). Those tests are pragmatic, can be used in any setting and their administration requires no special equipment. However, both tests rely on clinical judgement and the value of cut-off values for the TUG (>12, 14, 20 s?) and the turn 180° test are not well defined. The one leg stand test (less than 5 s?) has the same limits [8].

Other tests—such as the Berg balance test (useful in identifying the elders with low fall risk), the Tinetti scale, the functional reach and the dynamic gait test—may offer more detailed assessment and are of better diagnostic value, but they take longer to administer and need both equipment and clinical expertise [8].

Patients who stop walking when starting a conversation with a companion (dual task) are more prone to falls. People with a difference of 4.5 s or more between the TUG test (simple task) and the dual manual task TUG test (TUG test while carrying a glass of water in one hand) or who need 14.7 s or over to perform the cognitive TUG (TUG test while counting backward from a random start point) are at high risk of falling, especially in case of Parkinson's disease [9].

15.3.3 Tests to Assess Muscle Strength

These tests were well explained in the chapter focused on sarcopenia. The STEADI algorithm recommends using TUG, the 30-s chair stand, and the 4-stage balance test to identify people with gait/strength/balance disturbances (https://www.cdc.gov/steadi/index.html).

15.3.4 Composite Tests

The Short Physical Performance Battery (SPPB), that includes sit-to-stand performance, walking speed, and balance performance, demonstrates a significant association with fall history [10].

The Physiological Profile Assessment (PPA) that involves a series of simple tests of vision, peripheral sensation, muscle force, reaction time, postural sway, and the Timed up and go test can also be used to identify people at risk for falls [11].

As indicated previously, the above questions and tests should be particularly considered in patients with multimorbidity that may induce falls, including vision and cognitive impairment, incontinence, depression, and polypharmacy [12].

15.4 Profile of People Who Should Be Offered a Multifactorial Falls Risk Assessment

The 2013 NICE guidelines recommend that older people who present for medical attention because of a fall, or report recurrent falls in the past year, or demonstrate abnormalities of gait and/or balance when using above tests should be considered at sufficiently high risk of falling to be offered a multifactorial falls risk assessment [8]. With a slightly different approach, the American STEADI guidelines considers that people at high risk of falling are those with gait, strength or balance problems and with an history of injurious or recurrent falls (see above).

In subjects at low or moderate risk of falls, a multifactorial falls risk assessment is not needed; these persons should be proposed vitamin D ± calcium supplements, education, and be referred for strength and balance exercises (community exercise or fall prevention programme in case of low or moderate risk or physiotherapy in case of moderate risk of fall) (https://www.cdc.gov/steadi/pdf/STEADI-Algorithm-print.pdf).

15.5 Individualized Fall Interventions for Community-Dwelling Older Subjects

The NICE recommends that individualized multifactorial assessment and intervention should be performed by healthcare professionals with appropriate skills and experience, normally in the setting of a specialist falls service with clinic-level quality improvement strategies (e.g. case management), multifactorial assessment and treatment (e.g. comprehensive geriatric assessment) [8].

Factors to check in the STEADI multifactorial risk assessment include postural dizziness and postural hypotension, medication review, cognitive screening, use of mobility aids, feet and footwear, and visual acuity.

In addition to the management of causes and recognized risk factors of falls (of gait, balance and mobility disturbances, muscle weakness, and urinary incontinence), successful multifactorial intervention programmes comprise [8]:

15.5.1 Exercise Programmes [8, 13–18]

Group and home-based exercise programmes that combine balance and moderate intensity strength training either alone or with other interventions, including vision assessment and treatment, or environmental assessment and modification, are effective to prevent falls. The Otago, LIFE, Ossebo, and Falls Management Exercise (FaME) programmes have been demonstrated to reduce falls in older people at moderate or high risk of falling. Exercises to improve floor-rise ability and dual-task training should be included in clinical practice. There is no evidence that walking or brisk walking reduces the risk of falling. The NICE recommends that the exercise programme should be individually prescribed and monitored by an appropriately trained professional. The NICE guidelines recommend promoting the participation of older people in falls prevention programmes, considering the psychological and social values of such exercise programmes in addition to their physical benefits.

15.5.2 Home Hazard Intervention

The majority of fall-related injuries occur while older people move around home. Interventions to improve home safety, such as nightlights or bathroom grab bars, appear to be effective to reduce falls, especially in people at higher risk of falling, i.e. those who fall at home or have received treatment in hospital following a fall [8]. Home hazard interventions appear more effective when carried out by suitably trained healthcare professionals, especially occupational therapists [15]. NICE guidelines recommend promoting design modifications to the home by facilitating home visits by Information and Communication Technologies (ICT) specialists who could provide more sophisticated prevention and detection solutions [8].

15.5.3 Modification/Progressive Withdrawal of Fall Risk-Increasing Drugs (FRIDs)

Polypharmacy is a risk of falling. The most common FRIDs are—psychotropic drugs (sedatives, hypnotics, antidepressants, antipsychotic medications, antiepileptic, opioids, and other drugs which can cause sedation, delirium, or impaired balance and coordination—cardiovascular drugs and other drugs which can cause hyponatremia or worsen orthostatic hypotension (such as anticholinergic drugs) and induce cardiac arrhythmias. Those FRIDs are risk factors for injurious falls. A meta-analysis of randomized controlled interventions aiming to prevent falls in the elders living in the community reduces significantly the risk of falling by slow withdrawal of psychotropic and de-prescribing programmes [15, 19].

15.5.4 Cardiac Pacing

Insertion of a pacemaker should be considered for older people with frequent falls associated with cardio-inhibitory carotid sinus hypersensitivity, a condition which causes sudden changes in heart rate and blood pressure [8, 15].

15.5.5 Vision Optimization

Cataract surgery on the first affected eye and replacement of multifocal glasses by single lens glasses are effective in reducing the falling rate in older people living in the community [15]. Vision assessment and referral has been a component of successful multifactorial falls prevention programmes, especially when associated with home hazard intervention [8, 15]. Any history of cataracts, macular degeneration, glaucoma, or visual loss should be identified in people at risk of falling and those people should be referred to an eye doctor when no eye examination has occurred during the past year.

15.5.6 Osteoporosis Risk and Vitamin D

The STEADI guidelines recommend giving vitamin D and calcium supplementation in all patients, whatever their risk of falling [15, 20].

The NICE and more recent European guidelines recommend to perform a BMD and calculate the FRAX risk in patients at high risk of fall in order to determine recommendations for osteoporosis treatment [5, 21]. The prevalence of osteoporosis is high in patients who fall, especially in case of sarcopenia [22] (see chapter on this specific topic).

15.5.7 Multifaceted Podiatry

One trial conducted in 305 participants has shown that multifaceted podiatry, and foot and ankle exercises reduce significantly the rate of falls in people with disabling foot pains [15].

15.5.8 Encouraging Falls Prevention Programmes

Interventions that aim to increase knowledge/education about fall prevention alone seem not to be able to reduce significantly the rate of falls [15]. However, the NICE guidelines recommend implementing measures to enhance "fall awareness" in older people and healthcare professionals [8]. The American STEADI group recommends education in all older people and healthcare professionals (https://www.cdc.gov/steadi/materials.html). The Prevention of Falls Network for Dissemination (ProFouND) that is an European Commission funded initiative dedicated to the dissemination and implementation of best practice in fall prevention across Europe has also produced documents to influence policy and increase awareness of falls for health and social care authorities, the commercial sector, NGOs, and the general public (http://profound.eu.com/).

15.5.9 Public Environment

NICE guidelines recommend promoting design modifications of public environments, including "age-friendly" transportation modifications (NICE-2013).

On the whole, dedicated falls prevention programmes conducted in people living in the community decrease falls and fall-related injury rates by 20–40% and are cost effective [14, 15].

15.6 Fall Assessment in Care Settings

15.6.1 Fall Assessment in Inpatients

The 2016 NICE guidelines do not recommend to use fall risk prediction tools to assess inpatients' risk of falling in hospital but rather to consider that all hospitalized geriatric patients as well as younger patients judged by a clinician to be at significant risk of falling [8]. However, the St. Thomas risk assessment tool in falling elderly inpatients (STRATIFY) which assesses 5 factors (patients hospitalized for fall, visually impaired, agitated patients, patients who has fallen in the care facility since admission and patients with poor transfer and mobility in need of frequent toileting) has demonstrated a good sensitivity (93%) and specificity (88%) [23]. This scale appears not to be useful in patients undergoing geriatric rehabilitation [24]. The Hendrich II Fall Risk Model (HFRM) consists of 8 variables including confusion/disorientation/impulsivity, symptomatic depression, altered elimination, dizziness/vertigo, gender (female = 0, male = 1), any administered anti-epileptics, benzodiazepines, and the "get up and go" test (0–4). That instrument that needs only 3–5 min to complete has a high sensitivity and specificity to predict the risk of falling in hospital when used with a cut-off of 5 points [25].

15.6.2 Fall Assessment in Nursing Home Residents

Most of nursing home residents are at high risk of falling and risk assessment tools do not add significant value to nurses' judgement for identifying individuals at high risk of falls in daily practice [26].

15.7 Fall Interventions in Care Settings

15.7.1 Fall Interventions in Inpatients

The evidence for effective falls prevention interventions in acute and subacute wards is limited [27]. However, a recent randomized controlled trial showed that individualized patient education programmes, combined with training and feedback to staff, added to usual care, is effective to reduce the rates of falls and injurious falls in older patients in rehabilitation hospital-units [28]. This result confirms that regular practical face-to-face education and training for nurses, provision of equipment, audit, reminders and feedback, and the provision of falls data seem to be key factors to successful falls prevention programme implementation in inpatients [29]. NICE guidelines endorse the need to better understand which environmental improvements are the most effective and efficient for preventing falls and injuries in hospital. Architects should take into account these information when designing new hospitals [8].

15.7.2 Fall Interventions in Nursing Home Residents

Numerous types of interventions for nursing home residents have been tested, but it remains uncertain if these interventions have an effect on the rate of falls or the number of fallers [27]. Fall prevention interventions may however reduce the number of recurrent fallers [3]. The international evidence suggests that physical restraints may increase the risk of falling by constraining mobility in this group of frail elderly persons [30]. Educational programmes for all nursing staff (especially head nurses), residents, relatives, and legal guardians are effective to reduce physical restraint in nursing home residents [31].

15.8 Falls Clinics

Falls clinics are one approach by which older people with high levels of falls risk can be managed. Falls clinics that are however seldom in the world offer detailed multidisciplinary assessment and make recommendations or implement a range of targeted falls and falls injury-prevention strategies based on the assessment findings. Several pre–post clinic intervention studies and randomized controlled studies have indicated between 30 and 77% reductions in falls and related injuries in high falls risk populations. Moreover it was noticed improvements in other outcomes such as balance and mobility, physical functioning, fear of falling, and engagement with falls prevention interventions. The number of fallers that need to be treated in a fall clinic for one of them to avoid an injurious fall is estimated to be 5–6 [32].

Conclusion

Falls are a major public health problem in the ageing population. Some simple questions related to fall history in the previous months, feeling of unsteadiness, and fear of falling, and some simple tests aiming to assess balance/gait and muscle strength (timed up and go and sit-to-stand tests for example) may help to distinguish people at low, moderate, and high risk of falling. Strength and balance exercises are effective to reduce falls in people whatever the risk of falls. A multifactorial falls risk assessment and prevention should be offered to older people at high risk of falls, i.e. those who present for medical attention because of a fall, recurrent falls in the past year, or demonstrate abnormalities of gait and/or balance. This multifactorial falls risk assessment and prevention should be offered programme by a healthcare professional with appropriate skills and experience, normally in the setting of a falls clinic. Individualized, targeted multifactorial interventions comprise the management of specific causes of gait/balance and muscle strength disturbances, prescription of vitamin D supplements, measures to improve home safety (at best delivered by an occupational therapist), a review of medications, vision optimization, insertion of a pacemaker in case of carotid sinus hypersensitivity, and multifaceted podiatry. Because falls are most often preventable, it is now crucial to overcome limited awareness and usage of solutions to prevent and monitor falls and make these available [Action Group A2 of the European Innovation Partnership on Active and Healthy Ageing (EIP on AHA)] (https://ec.europa.eu/eip/ageing/action-group/index/a2_en).

References

1. Falls among older adults in the EU-28: key facts from the available statistics. https://eupha.org/repository/sections/ipsp/Factsheet_falls_in_older_adults_in_EU.pdf
2. Rapp K, Becker C, Cameron ID et al (2012) Epidemiology of falls in residential aged care: analysis of more than 70,000 falls from residents of bavarian nursing homes. J Am Med Dir Assoc 13:187.e1–187.e6
3. Vlaeyen E, Coussement J, Leysens G et al (2015) Center of Expertise for fall and fracture prevention Flanders. Characteristics and effectiveness of fall prevention programs in nursing homes: a systematic review and meta-analysis of randomized controlled trials. J Am Geriatr Soc 63:211–221
4. Krauss MJ, Evanoff B, Hitcho E et al (2005) A case–control study of patient, medication, and care-related risk factors for inpatient falls. J Gen Intern Med 20:116–122
5. Hanley A, Silke C, Murphy J (2011) Community-based health efforts for the prevention of falls in the elderly. Clin Interv Aging 6:19–25
6. Hartholt KA, Polinder S, Van der Cammen TJ et al (2012) Costs of falls in an ageing population: a nationwide study from the Netherlands (2007-2009). Injury 43:1199–1203

7. Phelan EA, Mahoney JE, Voit JC et al (2015) Assessment and management of fall risk in primary care settings. Med Clin North Am 99:281–293
8. https://www.nice.org.uk/guidance/cg161
9. Vance RC, Healy DG, Galvin R et al (2015) Dual tasking with the timed "up & go" test improves detection of risk of falls in people with Parkinson disease. Phys Ther 95:95–102
10. Kim JC, Chon J, Kim HS et al (2017) The association between fall history and physical performance tests in the community-dwelling elderly: a cross-sectional analysis. Ann Rehabil Med 41:239–247
11. Lord SR, Menz BH, Tiedemann A (2003) A physiological profile approach to falls risk assessment and prevention. Phys Ther 83:237–252
12. Stevens JA (2013) The STEADI tool kit: a fall prevention resource for health care providers. IHS Prim Care Provid 39:162–166
13. Rimland JM, Abraha I, Dell'Aquila G et al (2016) Effectiveness of non-pharmacological interventions to prevent falls in older people: a systematic overview. The SENATOR Project ONTOP Series. PLoS One 11:e0161579
14. Tricco AC, Thomas SM, Veroniki AA et al (2017) Comparisons of interventions for preventing falls in older adults: a systematic review and meta-analysis. JAMA 318:1687–1699
15. Gillespie LD, Robertson MC, Gillespie WJ et al (2012) Interventions for preventing falls in older people living in the community. Cochrane Database Syst Rev 9:CD007146
16. Huang ZG, Feng YH, Li YH et al (2017) Systematic review and meta-analysis: Tai Chi for preventing falls in older adults. BMJ Open 7:e013661
17. Hofmeyer MR, Alexander NB, Nyquist LV et al (2002) Floor-rise strategy training in older adults. J Am Geriatr Soc 50:1702–1706
18. Strouwen C, Molenaar EALM, Münks L et al (2017) Training dual tasks together or apart in Parkinson's disease: results from the DUALITY trial. Mov Disord 32:1201–1210
19. Musich S, Wang SS, Ruiz J et al (2017) Falls-related drug use and risk of falls among older adults: a study in a US Medicare population. Drugs Aging 34:555–565
20. Dhaliwal R, Aloia JF (2017) Effect of vitamin D on falls and physical performance. Endocrinol Metab Clin N Am 46:919–933
21. Blain H, Rolland Y, Beauchet O et al (2014) Usefulness of bone density measurement in fallers. Joint Bone Spine 81:403–408
22. Blain H, Masud T, Dargent-Molina P et al (2016) A comprehensive fracture prevention strategy in older adults: the European Union Geriatric Medicine Society (EUGMS) statement. Eur Geriatr Med 7:519–525
23. Davis JC, Robertson MC, Ashe MC et al (2010) International comparison of cost of falls in older adults living in the community: a systematic review. Osteoporos Int 21:1295–1306
24. Aranda-Gallardo M, Morales-Asencio JM, Canca-Sanchez JC et al (2013) Instruments for assessing the risk of falls in acute hospitalized patients: a systematic review and meta-analysis. BMC Health Serv Res 13:122
25. Zhang C, Wu X, Lin S et al (2015) Evaluation of reliability and validity of the Hendrich II fall risk model in a Chinese hospital population. PLoS One 6:e0142395
26. Holte HH, Underland V, Hafstad E. et al (2015) Review of systematic reviews on prevention of falls in Institutions NIPH Systematic Reviews: Executive Summaries Report from Norwegian Knowledge Centre for the Health Services. p 13
27. Cameron ID, Gillespie LD, Robertson MC et al (2012) Interventions for preventing falls in older people in care facilities and hospitals. Cochrane Database Syst Rev 12:CD005465
28. Hill AM, McPhail SM, Waldron N et al (2015) Fall rates in hospital rehabilitation units after individualised patient and staff education programmes: a pragmatic, stepped-wedge, cluster-randomised controlled trial. Lancet 385:2592–2599
29. Ayton DR, Barker AL, Morello RT et al (2017) Barriers and enablers to the implementation of the 6-PACK falls prevention program: a pre-implementation study in hospitals participating in a cluster randomised controlled trial. PLoS One 12:e0171932
30. Morley JE (2010) Clinical practice in nursing homes as a key for progress. J Nutr Health Aging 14:586–593

31. Köpke S, Mühlhauser I, Gerlach A et al (2012) Effect of a guideline-based multicomponent intervention on use of physical restraints in nursing homes: a randomized controlled trial. JAMA 307:2177–2184
32. Palvanen M, Kannus P, Piirtola M et al (2014) Effectiveness of the Chaos Falls Clinic in preventing falls and injuries of home-dwelling older adults: a randomised controlled trial. Injury 45:265–271

Promotion of a Lifelong Immunization Program for Healthy Ageing

16

Johan Flamaing

Key Messages

- Adult vaccination is often neglected in midlife.
- Later in life, multimorbidity, frailty, malnutrition, and immunosenescence increase the risk of vaccine preventable diseases.
- Due to worldwide vaccination, tetanus and diphtheria became rare diseases. In Europe, tetanus and diphtheria affect mainly older adults with a high mortality rate.
- Pertussis is a frequent disease in adults (parents and grandparents), with regular transmission to children.
- Excess winter mortality in persons 65+ can be attributed to influenza and low vaccine coverages in this target population and their (in)formal caregivers.
- The mortality rate of invasive pneumococcal disease is highest in older persons and 60 times higher for persons 85+ than for children.
- The incidence of shingles and postherpetic neuralgia increases with age with a subsequent negative impact on quality of life.
- There is a suboptimal protection against these vaccine preventable diseases (VPDs).
- A lifelong vaccination strategy that directly (vaccination and boosting) and indirectly (herd protection) protects against VPD is the best option to optimally protect older adults.
- Vaccine providers and the healthcare system must coordinate their efforts to increase vaccine uptake from birth till old age.

J. Flamaing
Department of Geriatric Medicine, UZ Leuven, Leuven, Belgium

Division of Gerontology and Geriatrics, Department of Chronic Diseases, Metabolism, and Ageing (CHROMETA), KU Leuven, Leuven, Belgium
e-mail: johan.flamaing@uzleuven.be

J.-P. Michel (ed.), *Prevention of Chronic Diseases and Age-Related Disability*, Practical Issues in Geriatrics, https://doi.org/10.1007/978-3-319-96529-1_16

16.1 Introduction

The burden of infectious diseases is spread throughout life but young children and older adults mostly have the highest incidence, morbidity, and mortality caused by infections.

In infants immunity needs to be acquired to cope with infections later in life and in many countries immunization against vaccine preventable diseases (VPDs) is embedded in national childhood vaccination programs supported by the healthcare system, GPs, child care and school prevention programs.

For adults, unless there is an occupational hazard for a VPD with an associated prevention program in the workplace, the individual person is often responsible for his/her immunization.

In the older age group, a complex and heterogeneous population regarding multimorbidity, frailty, cognitive and physical function, and nutritional status, the risk and consequences of VPD are most pronounced but a structured approach to VPD prevention in this population is often lacking.

In this chapter, the rationale and impact of a lifelong vaccination program that helps attaining the goal of "healthy ageing" is discussed.

16.2 Vaccine Preventable Disease Epidemiology in Older Persons

The incidence and impact (morbidity, mortality) of relevant VPD that affect (older) adults are summarized in this section.

16.2.1 Tetanus

With an estimated global Tetanus-diphtheria (Td) vaccination coverage of nearly 90%, tetanus has become a rare disease with 13,502 reported cases worldwide in 2016. Neonatal tetanus is estimated to cause the death of 61,000 newborns yearly (2011) mainly in rural areas with poor perinatal hygiene [1]. In developed countries, where tetanus has become a rare disease, its incidence is highest in the older population, increases with advancing age and mortality is five times higher than in the population under 65 years reaching a mortality rate of 50% for persons over 80 years [2].

This higher incidence in older persons is correlated with a lower vaccine coverage in the population over 65 years (50% in the article referred) and the lack of protective levels of antibodies in about 70% of persons 70 years or older [3].

16.2.2 Diphtheria

Due to the combined vaccination against tetanus and diphtheria, the latter VPD has also become rare with 7079 cases reported globally in 2016 [4]. In the EU, 35 cases were reported in 2014 (22 C. diphtheriae and 13 C. ulcerans cases). Diphtheria occurred in every age groups, 11% in persons 65 years or older and one lethal case occurred in an 88 years old woman. Vaccination coverage in the diphtheria cases was only 50%. A lack of protective diphtheria antitoxin immunoglobulins has been shown in up to 70% of the older population [5].

16.2.3 Pertussis

An increasing incidence of pertussis is reported worldwide (2016: 139,535 reported cases) and in the EU (40,727 cases in 2014, a 2.5-fold increase compared to 2000). Waning immunity, awareness, and better diagnostics can explain this increase [6].

Vaccination strategies for pertussis: vaccination of newborns, infants, children, healthcare workers (HCW), pregnant women, adults, and cocoon vaccination aim to protect young infants, while disease burden in the (older) adult population is underestimated due to an often asymptomatic or mild course.

However, passive surveillance and outbreak data suggest that up to 58% of pertussis cases occur in persons 60 years or older resulting in hospitalizations with a longer length of stay (LOS) and deaths (often by cerebral hemorrhage) [7].

In pertussis cases, 44% are un- or under vaccinated [6]. Only 22% of persons 65 years or older reported being vaccinated against pertussis the last 10 years in the USA [8]. Protective immunity against pertussis wanes after 5–10 years. Although no good correlate for protection exists for pertussis, 1/3 adults had no detectable antibodies against pertussis despite childhood vaccination in an Australian and Belgian population, suggesting susceptibility to the disease [9].

16.2.4 Influenza

The yearly influenza epidemics result in a disproportionally high burden of disease in older persons with great inter-seasonal variation depending on the circulating influenza strain (with a higher burden in older persons for H3N2 > H1N1 > B).

While the rates of influenza-related GP visits are not highest in the older population (the highest rate of GP visits is in children), the rates for influenza-related hospitalizations, ICU admissions and deaths are. In the older population the presence of chronic conditions more than doubles the influenza-related hospitalization rate, while mortality is comparable with or without risk condition (chronic obstructive respiratory disease, cardiovascular, central nervous system, renal and liver disorders, diabetes, immunosuppressive conditions, or stroke) [10]. In Europe, 88% of the excess winter mortality in persons 65 years or older could be attributed to the H3N2 epidemic in 2016–2017 [11].

Although vaccination against influenza is recommended for older persons and persons at risk in most European countries, the EU goal of 75% coverage of the target population was only reached in three countries for the season 2012–2013 (The Netherlands, UK Northern Ireland, and UK Scotland) [12]. Decreasing trends in influenza vaccine coverage are documented in several countries (Belgium and Italy) [13, 14].

16.2.5 Pneumococcal Disease

While the incidence of (invasive) pneumococcal disease (IPD) is highest in children, mortality of IPD is concentrated in older persons. With an overall mortality rate of 1/100,000, the IPD mortality in persons 85 years or older (11.56/100,000) is nearly 60 times higher than in children (0.2/100,000). Every decade after the age of 50, the mortality rate of IPD doubles from 1.5/100,000 for the age group 50–64 to the mortality rate for persons 85 years or older mentioned above [15].

WHO does not prioritize adult pneumococcal vaccination [16]. Pneumococcal vaccination of older adults, although recommended in the majority of European countries and the USA, is not well established in most of these countries. The best PPV23 uptake is documented in England with an uptake of 70% in persons 65 years or older and reaching just over 80% in persons 75 years or older [17]. Vaccination with PPV23, PCV 13, or both vaccines was only reported by 43%, 31.5%, and 18.3% of Medicare beneficiaries belonging to the target group for pneumococcal vaccination, respectively, despite the Advisory Committee on Immunization Practices (ACIP, USA) recommendation to use both vaccines sequentially [18]. In Belgium, only 12.5% of persons 75 years of age reported being vaccinated with a decreasing trend over time and the Netherlands does not recommend pneumococcal vaccination in adults [14].

16.2.6 Herpes Zoster (HZ)

The incidence of herpes zoster increases with age and is four times higher in persons 95 years and older (9.45/1000 person years) than in persons of 40 years (2.15/1000 person years. Mainly hospitalization-based diagnoses for HZ increase substantially with advancing age (with a factor 10 between 40 and 90 years (0.1 to 1.1/1000 person years). Sixty percent of HZ diagnoses are made in women and depending upon the severity, immunosuppression can double HZ incidence rates [19]. Due to population ageing and extended life expectancy, a 100–300% increase of HZ cases is expected depending on the country's demography. The incidence of postherpetic neuralgia, the most common complication of HZ infection, and its duration, also increases with age. Postherpetic neuralgia (PHN) has an impact on the quality of life in all health domains [20].

Vaccination against HZ and PHN is recommended since 2008 in the USA and in the UK since 2010. In the USA, 31% of persons 65 years or older were vaccinated against HZ in 2014 and in the UK 55% of persons 70 or 78 years of age were vaccinated in 2015, but the vaccination coverage was dropping compared to previous years [8]. Other countries (Germany, France, Belgium) also developed guidelines for vaccination against HZ but data on vaccine uptake are lacking.

All these data demonstrate the high burden of and suboptimal protection against VPD in the (older) adult population. In persons 65 years or over more than 5, 2 million VPD (Influenza, Pneumococcal disease, Herpes Zoster, and Pertussis) cases occurred with an associated cost of more than 15 billion dollars in 2015 in the USA [21]. Even highly developed countries struggle to obtain a high vaccine uptake in older adults.

16.3 The Impact of Frailty, Immunosenescence, and Comorbidity on Vaccine Effect

Immunosenescence is the decline in systemic immunity associated with ageing and involves both innate and adaptive immune responses. Oligoclonal accumulation of senescent T-lymphocytes stimulated by latent (herpes) viruses with less naïve T-lymphocytes to combat new infections is a key feature in immunosenescence of the adaptive immune system. Therefore older adults are more susceptible to VPD that tend to be more severe than in younger people. Immunosenescence also impairs the capacity to respond to a vaccine with lower vaccine effectiveness as a consequence. While the primary immune response is blunted in older persons, the recall or booster response seems to be intact [22]. The elderly population is extremely heterogeneous with a variety of underlying medical conditions, medications, nutritional, functional and cognitive status, previous infections, and environmental exposures. In this complex phenotype, the isolation of the contribution of immunosenescence to VPD susceptibility and vaccine (in)effectiveness is difficult. In carefully selected healthy older persons, the immune responses to vaccines are comparable to younger adults. The correlation between the frailty syndrome, immunosenescence, and vaccine response/effect needs clarification, as immune response and effectiveness studies comparing frail, prefail, and fit older persons give conflicting results [23, 24].

16.3.1 Pneumococcal Vaccines

In contrast to the 2013 Cochrane review concluding that in high-risk elderly and adults with underlying conditions the 23-valent pneumococcal polysaccharide vaccine (PPV23) does not offer protection against pneumococcal disease, recent meta-analyses show that PPV23 protects against both invasive pneumococcal disease and pneumococcal pneumonia [25]. The 13-valent pneumococcal conjugate vaccine (PCV13) protects older adults with underlying conditions against IPD and pneumococcal pneumonia caused by PCV13 serotypes with an age dependent decline (VE 65% to VE 40% between 65 and 75 years) up to the age of 80 years [26]. PCV13 induces a boostable immune-memory with comparable or higher secondary serotype-specific antibodies. Combining the effectiveness of PCV13 and broad coverage of PPV23 may offer older adults the best protection against pneumococcal disease (pneumococcal pneumonia and invasive disease).

16.3.2 Influenza Vaccine

Older persons are able to mount protective levels of antibodies against influenza virus. No difference in seroprotection was found between institutionalized persons 60–85 years and persons >85 years in an analysis of immunogenicity data over 21 seasons in Italy for 2 of the 3 strains (except B) in the trivalent inactivated influenza vaccine (TIV). Women, new antigens and enhanced (adjuvanted or intradermally (ID)) vaccines mounted a better response irrespective of age [27].

Controversy on the protective effect of TIV in the elderly persists and is mainly caused by the lack of adequately powered RCTs in this population and the biases present in observational studies where different inclusion criteria, settings, and outcomes are reported. However, recent studies show that TIV prevents lab confirmed influenza (VE: 42–54%), hospitalizations (VE: 40–47%), and mortality (VE: 16%, NNV: 65–74 years: 649, ≥75 years: 251) in older persons and that the level of protection is influenced by age, comorbid conditions, and influenza type (protection against H1N1 > B > H3N2) [28, 29].

16.3.3 Herpes Zoster Vaccine (VZV)

The live-attenuated VZV reduces the overall incidence of VZ (VE: 51.3%), PHN (VE: 66.5%), and the burden of illness (BOI) related to VZ (VE: 61.1%). These effects are age and time dependent. In higher age groups, the VE on HZ incidence is less (60–69 years: 64%, 70–79 years: 41%), and no significant VE was present in persons 80 years or older. This age dependent VE decline was not demonstrated for PHN and BOI but data on VE ≥ 80 years were not available in the Shingles Prevention Study (SPS). The VE also wanes over time. In long-term follow-up studies of the SPS (up to 11 years after vaccination), a decline in VE for HZ incidence (VE: 51.3% to 31.1% in year 8 of FU), BOI (VE: 61.1% to 33.3% in year 10 of FU), and PHN (VE: 66.5% to 35.4%) was noticed. Whether revaccination could be beneficial needs further evaluation [30].

An inactivated adjuvanted subunit VZV in a 2 dose schedule demonstrated a VE of ±90% on the incidence of HZ and PHN even in persons ≥80 years. FDA/EMA approval for this vaccine has been obtained [31].

16.3.4 Tetanus, Diphtheria, and Pertussis (Tdap) Vaccine

The level of antibodies protective against tetanus, diphtheria, and pertussis wane over time. Booster vaccination is recommended every 10 years. Older persons ≥65 years mount a good booster antibody response against tetanus (94.5% seroprotection), diphtheria (82.8% seroprotection), and pertussis antigens (±90% seroprotection depending on the antigen) [32].

There are no trials on the effectiveness of Tdap vaccination in older persons because high coverage rates have made clinical VPD rare (see section on epidemiology of tetanus, diphtheria, and pertussis).

16.4 Strategies to Augment Protection of Older Persons Against VPD

Enhanced protection of older persons against VPD can be achieved by the use of more efficient vaccines, vaccination strategies, and vaccine implementation.

16.4.1 Augmenting the Vaccine Effect

As immune-rejuvenation to combat immunosenescence is at this moment not possible, the use of more immunogenic vaccine formulations in older persons is a good choice to better protect older persons against VPD.

Vaccines that induce a higher immune response (and possibly better protection against VPD) are to be preferred in older persons. For this purpose, higher doses of antigens in vaccines (e.g., TIV), adjuvanted vaccines (e.g., MF59 adjuvanted TIV, adjuvanted VZV), specific vaccine formulations (e.g., virosomal vs. split virus inactivated TIV, pneumococcal conjugate vs. polysaccharide vaccine, live-attenuated vs. conjugated HZV), and applications (e.g., intradermal vs. sc TIV) induce higher protective antibody levels.

Vaccines must protect against circulating epidemic strains and adaptation of vaccine formulations is often necessary. Yearly adaptation of influenza vaccines with broader coverage (e.g., QIV (H1N1, H3N2, B Yamagata, and B Victoria) vs. TIV (without B Victoria) will have higher protective potential depending on the circulating strains of influenza. A mismatch can lead to higher influenza related disease burden and mortality. Including more (prevalent) pneumococcal serotypes in pneumococcal vaccines will broaden the protection against pneumococcal disease (PCV 7—PCV 13—PPV 23).

Boosting immune-memory after priming vaccination can maintain antibodies and protection against VPD. Repeat vaccination is necessary to protect against tetanus, diphtheria, pertussis, and influenza. Using the pneumococcal polysaccharide or conjugate vaccine after priming with the pneumococcal conjugate vaccine induces a booster response. Whether repeat vaccination over time with pneumococcal and HZ vaccines is beneficial is not clearly established [33].

16.4.2 Vaccination Strategies

Age-based vaccination (childhood vaccination program, vaccination of persons 60–65 years or older), occupational vaccination (HCW, occupational exposition (e.g., poultry farmers)), and risk-based vaccination (for chronic diseases and/or immunocompromising conditions) are strategies that aim at protecting susceptible persons directly against VPD.

While the strategies mentioned above augment direct protection, an indirect protection of older persons against VPD can be obtained by vaccinating the population serving as an important reservoir and/or vector for VPD. Persons lacking protection against VPD have a lower chance contracting a VPD when most of the population susceptible to the VPD is vaccinated (herd protection). Vaccinating children (and adults) against influenza protects the older population against influenza and influenza-related hospitalization and mortality. This resulted in the recommendation to vaccinate all citizens in the USA against influenza [34]. Vaccination of children against pneumococcal disease resulted in a significant decline of the incidence and mortality caused by invasive pneumococcal disease in the USA in the older

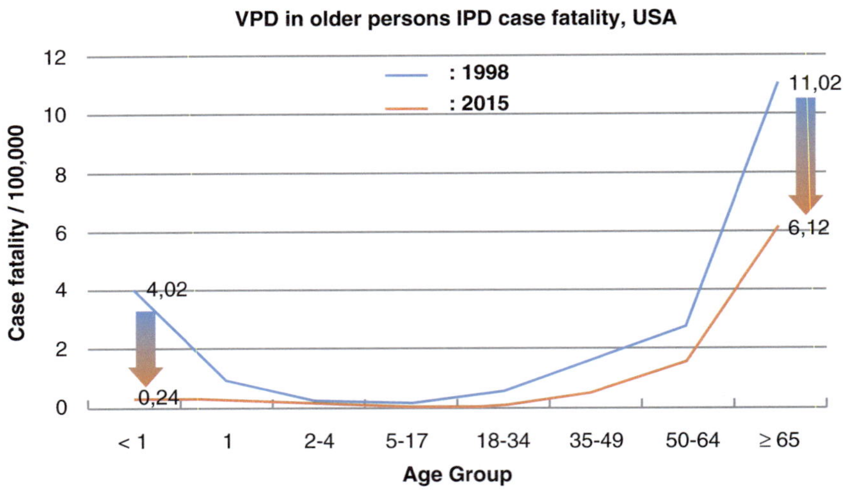

Fig. 16.1 Case fatality of invasive pneumococcal disease in the USA 1998 vs. 2015. *VPD* vaccine preventable disease, *IPD* invasive pneumococcal disease

population as well (Fig. 16.1, [15]). Vaccination against pertussis should be maintained throughout life (cocoon vaccination) not only for direct protection, but also to reduce transmission to the very young and very old.

Caregivers and HCWs in contact with older persons can protect themselves against VPD (hepatitis A and B, influenza, tetanus, diphtheria, and pertussis). Additionally transmission of VPD from themselves towards susceptible persons is prevented.

Taking all these considerations together vaccination should be considered as a tool to prevent VPD throughout life and not only for certain age- or risk-groups. A lifelong vaccination program incorporating direct (priming and boosting vaccination) and indirect (herd) protection against VPD in a lifelong vaccination program is the best strategy to obtain (VPD free) healthy ageing. As an example, the scheme of Italian lifelong vaccination program is shown in Fig. 16.2 [35].

16.4.3 Vaccine Implementation

Despite the high burden of VPD in (older) adults and the availability of effective vaccines, the vaccine uptake in this population is often very low in many countries (cf. VPD epidemiology section of this article).

Il calendario vaccinale del Piano Nazionale di Prevenzione Vaccinale 2017-2019

Vaccino	0gg-30gg	3° mese	4° mese	5° mese	6° mese	7° mese	11° mese	13° mese	15° mese	6° anno	12°-18° anno	19-49 anni	50-64 anni	> 64 anni	Soggetti ad anumentato rischio
DTPa**		DTPa		DTPa			DTPa			DTPa**	dTpaIPV	1 dose dTpa**** ogni 10 anni			(1)
IPV		IPV		IPV			IPV			IPV					
Epatite B	EpB-EpB*	Ep B		Ep B			Ep B								(2)
Hib		Hib		Hib			Hib								(3)
Pneumococco		PCV		PCV			PCV							PCV+PPSV	(4) ^^
MPRV								MPRV		MPRV					(6) ^
MPR								oppure MPR		oppure MPR					(5)*****
Varicella								+ V		+ V					(6)^
Meningococco C								Men C[5]			Men ACWY coniugato				(7)
Meningococco B*^		Men B	Men B		Men B			Men B							
HPV											HPV°: 2-3 dosi (in funzione di età e vaccino)				(8)
Influenza														1 dose all'anno	(9)°°
Herpes Zoster														1 dose#	(10)
Rotavirus		Rotavirus## (due o tre dosi a seconda del tipo di vaccino)													
Epatite A															(11)

Fig. 16.2 National lifelong vaccination calendar, Italy 2017–2019. Vaccine abbreviations not translated from Italian

There are three parties involved in the implementation of vaccination: the vaccine recipient, the vaccine provider, and the healthcare system.

Active recommendation to be vaccinated by the primary healthcare professional is the most important factor that enhances vaccine uptake in the recipient besides awareness of personal disease risk for VPD, safety of vaccination, accessibility, and cost of vaccination. Household, family members and directives from healthcare institutions recommending vaccination support individual vaccination.

The knowledge of VPD and vaccine effects and positive (pay per performance) and/or negative (penalty/control via a vaccination threshold) incentives to vaccinate are the factors driving the vaccine providers willingness to vaccinate.

The healthcare system can, at different levels, do VPD surveillance, issue vaccination guidelines, raise awareness and knowledge of VPD and vaccination in recipients and providers, reimburse vaccine costs for recipients, and give incentives to providers.

There is a complex interplay between these three stakeholders and a multicomponent coordinated intervention framework is needed to have an impact on vaccine uptake (Fig. 16.3, [36]).

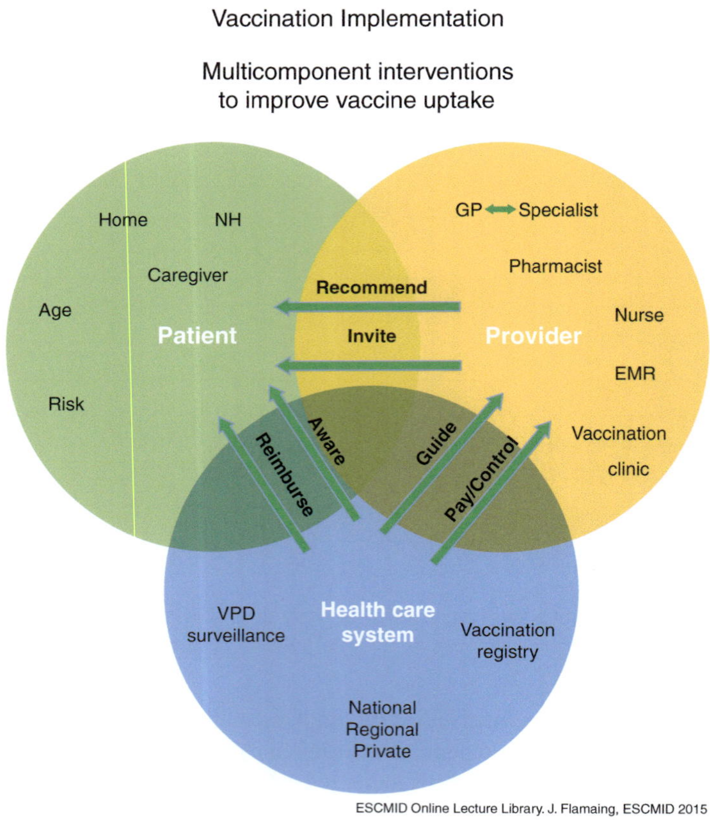

Fig. 16.3 Stakeholders and interventions in multicomponent interventions to improve vaccination implementation. *NH* nursing home, *GP* general physician, *EMR* electronic medical record, *VPD* vaccine preventable disease

Conclusion

A lifelong vaccination strategy that directly (vaccination and boosting) and indirectly (herd protection) protects against VPD by installing and maintaining specific immunity during a life course is the best option to optimally protect older adults. A multicomponent intervention that involves vaccinees, providers, and the healthcare system should be adopted by all countries to lower the burden of VPD and its associated costs.

References

1. World Health Organization (2017) http://www.who.int/immunization/monitoring_surveillance/burden/vpd/surveillance_type/passive/tetanus_coverage.jpg?ua=1. Accessed Sept 2017
2. Centers for Disease Control and Prevention (2011) VPD Surveillance Manual, 5th edn. Tetanus: Chapter 16–1. https://www.cdc.gov/vaccines/pubs/surv-manual/chpt16-tetanus.pdf. Accessed Sept 2017

3. Williams WW, Lu PJ, O'Halloran A et al (2015) Vaccination coverage among adults, excluding influenza vaccination—United States, 2013. MMWR Morb Mortal Wkly Rep 64:95–102
4. WHO immunization, vaccines and biologicals: Diphteria. http://www.who.int/immunization/monitoring_surveillance/burden/diphtheria/en/
5. Edmunds WJ, Pebody RG, Aggerback H et al (2000) The sero-epidemiology of diphtheria in Western Europe. ESEN Project. European Sero-Epidemiology Network. Epidemiol Infect 125:113–125
6. WHO immunization, vaccines and biologicals: Pertussis: http://www.who.int/immunization/monitoring_surveillance/burden/vpd/surveillance_type/passive/pertussis/en/
7. Ridda I, Yin JK, King C et al (2012) The importance of pertussis in older adults: a growing case for reviewing vaccination strategy in the elderly. Vaccine 30:6745–6752
8. Williams WW, Lu PJ, O'Halloran A et al (2017) Surveillance of vaccination coverage among adult populations—United States, 2015. MMWR Surveill Summ 66:1–28
9. Van Damme P, Burgess M (2004) Immunogenicity of a combined diphtheria-tetanus-acellular pertussis vaccine in adults. Vaccine 22:305–308
10. Fleming DM, Taylor RJ, Haguinet F et al (2016) Influenza-attributable burden in United Kingdom primary care. Epidemiol Infect 144:537–547
11. Vestergaard LS, Nielsen J, Krause TG et al (2017) Excess all-cause and influenza-attributable mortality in Europe, December 2016 to February 2017. Euro Surveill 22:30506. https://doi.org/10.2807/1560-7917.ES.2017.22.14.30506
12. ECDC technical report: seasonal influenza vaccination Europe 2012–13. https://ecdc.europa.eu/sites/portal/files/media/en/publications/Publications/Seasonal-influenza-vaccination-Europe-2012-13.pdf
13. Poscia A, Stojanovic J, Ricciardi W (2016) The sustainability of influenza vaccination programs: considerations and perspectives from Italy. J Prev Med Hyg 57:E9–E12
14. Wetenschappelijk Instituut Volksgezondheid, Gezondheidsenquête 2013, rapport 5: preventie. https://his.wiv-isp.be/nl/Gedeelde%20%20documenten/VA_NL_2013.pdf
15. Centers for Disease Control and Prevention (1998 to 2015) Active Bacterial Core Surveillance Report, Emerging Infections Program Network, *Streptococcus pneumoniae*
16. WHO (2012) Pneumococcal vaccines WHO position paper—2012. Wkly Epidemiol Rec 87:129–144 http://www.who.int/wer/2012/wer8714.pdf?ua=1
17. Public Health England (2017) Pneumococcal Polysaccharide Vaccine (PPV) coverage report, England, April 2016 to March 2017. Health Protect Rep 11:23 https://www.gov.uk/government/uploads/system/uploads/attachment_data/file/624133/hpr2317_PPV.pdf
18. Black CL, Williams WW, Warnock R et al (2017) Pneumococcal vaccination among Medicare beneficiaries occurring after the advisory committee on immunization practices recommendation for routine use of 13-valent pneumococcal conjugate vaccine and 23-valent pneumococcal polysaccharide vaccine for adults aged ≥65 years. MMWR Morb Mortal Wkly Rep 66:728–733
19. Schröder C, Enders D, Schink T et al (2017) Incidence of herpes zoster amongst adults varies by severity of immunosuppression. J Infect 75:207–215
20. Drolet M, Brisson M, Schmader KE et al (2010) The impact of herpes zoster and post-herpetic neuralgia on health-related quality of life: a prospective study. CMAJ 182:1731–1736
21. McLaughlin JM, McGinnis JJ, Tan L et al (2015) Estimated human and economic burden of four major adult vaccine-preventable diseases in the United States, 2013. J Prim Prev 36:259–273
22. Chen WH, Kozlovsky BF, Effros RB et al (2009) Vaccination in the elderly: an immunological perspective. Trends Immunol 30:351–359
23. Yao X, Hamilton RG, Weng NP et al (2011) Frailty is associated with impairment of vaccine-induced antibody response and increase in post-vaccination influenza infection in community-dwelling older adults. Vaccine 29:5015–5021
24. Van Epps P, Tumpey T, Pearce MB et al (2017) Preexisting immunity, not frailty phenotype, predicts influenza postvaccination titers among older veterans. Clin Vaccine Immunol 24:e00498

25. Falkenhorst G, Remschmidt C, Harder T et al (2017) Effectiveness of the 23-valent pneumococcal polysaccharide vaccine (PPV23) against pneumococcal disease in the elderly: systematic review and meta-analysis. PLoS One 12:e0169368
26. van Werkhoven CH, Huijts SM, Bolkenbaas M et al (2015) The impact of age on the efficacy of 13-valent pneumococcal conjugate vaccine in elderly. Clin Infect Dis 61:1835–1838
27. Nunzi E, Iorio AM, Camilloni B (2017) A 21-winter seasons retrospective study of antibody response after influenza vaccination in elderly (60-85 years old) and very elderly (>85 y.o.) institutionalized subjects. Hum Vaccin Immunother 13(11):2659–2668. https://doi.org/10.1080/21645515.2017.1373226
28. Jackson ML, Chung JR, Jackson LA et al (2017) Influenza vaccine effectiveness in the United States during the 2015-2016 season. N Engl J Med 377:534–543
29. Castilla J, Guevara M, Martínez-Baz I et al (2015) Enhanced estimates of the influenza vaccination effect in preventing mortality: a prospective cohort study. Medicine (Baltimore) 94:e1240
30. Oxman MN, Levin MJ, Johnson GR et al (2005) A vaccine to prevent herpes zoster and postherpetic neuralgia in older adults. N Engl J Med 352:2271–2284
31. Cunningham AL, Lal H, Kovac M et al (2016) Efficacy of the Herpes Zoster subunit vaccine in adults 70 years of age or older. N Engl J Med 375:1019–1032
32. Van Damme P, McIntyre P, Grimprel E et al (2011) Immunogenicity of the reduced-antigen-content dTpa vaccine (Boostrix(®)) in adults 55 years of age and over: a sub-analysis of four trials. Vaccine 29:5932–5939
33. Lang PO, Aspinall R (2014) Vaccination in the elderly: what can be recommended? Drugs Aging 31:581–589
34. Grohskopf LA, Sokolow LZ, Broder KR et al (2017) Prevention and control of seasonal influenza with vaccines: recommendations of the Advisory Committee on Immunization Practices—United States, 2017-18 Influenza Season. MMWR Recomm Rep 66:1–20
35. Bonanni P, Azzari C, Castiglia P et al (2014) The 2014 lifetime immunization schedule approved by the Italian scientific societies. Italian Society of Hygiene, Preventive Medicine, and Public Health. Italian Society of Pediatrics. Italian Federation of Pediatric Physicians. Italian Federation of General Medical Physicians. Arezzo Service of Legal Medicine. Epidemiol Prev 38:131–146
36. Bonanni P, Bonaccorsi G, Lorini C et al (2017) Focusing on the implementation of 21st century vaccines for adults. Vaccine. pii: S0264-410X(17)31036–8. [Epub ahead of print]. https://doi.org/10.1016/j.vaccine.2017.07.100

How Healthy Ageing Can Foster Age-Friendly Environment?

17

Suzanne Garon and Mario Paris

Key Messages

- Healthy ageing is an important framework that is conceived to help governmental bodies to address the long-term challenges of their ageing population.
- The built and social environments shall be taken into account to enhance the functional abilities of the new generation of seniors in all countries.
- Taking part in the age-friendly cities and communities world network could enhance government bodies to develop and implement new and low-cost strategies to face the challenges associated to their ageing population.

17.1 A Brief Historic Return of a Successful Concept

Active and healthy ageing are two distinct frameworks which require clarification due to their polysemy and because they are sometimes used interchangeably. Their meaning has gone through an evolution over the years which now make them more distinguishable. The following clarifications are based on the work of Moulaert, Boudiny and Paris [1]. Active ageing appeared in the 1990s as a junction of international organisations and social gerontologist concerns. Three general types of active ageing promote an ongoing participation of older adults in society and therefore, a divergence from a more traditional model of encouraging the withdrawal from society. The first type is a unidimensional approach (mainly participation in the labour

S. Garon (✉)
School of Social Work, Université de Sherbrooke, Quebec, QC, Canada

Research Center on Aging—CIUSSS de l'Estrie—CHUS, Sherbrooke, QC, Canada
e-mail: suzanne.garon@usherbrooke.ca

M. Paris
School of Social Work, Université de Moncton, Moncton, NB, Canada

J.-P. Michel (ed.), *Prevention of Chronic Diseases and Age-Related Disability*, Practical Issues in Geriatrics, https://doi.org/10.1007/978-3-319-96529-1_17

market or physical activity). The second type is a multidimensional approach (various areas of participation in a perspective of the continuation of activities previously done as an adult). Finally, the third type transcends the behavioural level to include health and economic conditions. Healthy ageing relies on three main principals: it is a global approach (a lifelong process of optimising, improving and preserving) with multiple dimensions (health, physical, social and mental wellness, independence, qualify of life and successful life-transition), it is based on social interactions (including in the workplace but also through volunteer activities, social activities, etc.), and it is both linked to the process of ageing as well as to old age. Both active ageing and healthy ageing have some limitations, such as the absence of recognising that ageing can be marked by decline, the individualisation of responsibility (which can lead to victim blaming for those who seem to be succeeding based on obscure or elitist social criteria), and a confusion of terms. "By considering health as a determinant of active ageing rather than a constituent – i.e. by conceiving health as a means to active aging, not the end- the common criticism to the active aging discourse…" (p. 290) has no consideration for the older adults incapable of reaching the goal due to physical, mental or social limitations [1].

17.2 Healthy Ageing, The 2015 Version

The WHO reintroduced the concept of healthy ageing in the 2015 World Report on Ageing and Health (WRAH) [2]. The objective was to promote a shift from active ageing, which had been used since 2002, to healthy ageing. The significance of the newer concept is the emphasis placed on a broader sense of health.

Nevertheless, many researchers in the field of the Age-Friendly Cities and Communities were extremely concerned about the effects of this new policy. Their apprehension was that healthy ageing may reduce ageing to merely a medical problem. Too often, ageing in our societies is considered only through the lens of a narrow medical perspective and in so doing, leads to two major limitations. Firstly, ageing is interpreted by the degrees of deterioration of health where there is little response besides providing medication as if treating a chronic disease. If it is urgent that every country should have specific care for this growing ageing population, it is equally as important that the social stigma on ageing be addressed as well. Otherwise, this medical trend provides a prejudicial portrait of the ageing population, where older adults are represented as a social burden and thereby increasing the effects of ageism. The second flaw is the individualisation of the responsibility of ageing. Ageing is a biological process that takes place in social contexts, more specifically in built and social environments. There is a fundamental link between the ageing process of any specific person and the society in which that person lives. As we saw in the work of Moulaert et al., the individualisation of the responsibility of ageing fuels social injustice. As Holstein and Minkler already noticed, "to make sure that we do not further marginalise the already marginalised, both individual and contextual factors need to be taken into account…" (p. 289) [1, 3]. In the WRHA, emphasis is placed on the importance of taking into account environments. Specifically, in relation to the "trajectory" and the concepts of functional ability, we will see further on.

The WRHA provides the opportunity for the WHO to enhance their relationships with the different health ministries around the world in order to increase interest on the subject of ageing. To put the focus on health corresponds also to the goal of shaping a worldwide agenda to address the reality of ageing and to offer a path to find solutions and innovation in providing services and care. Presented as a public-health framework, this document supports four priorities or areas where action has to be achieved:

1. Aligning health systems with the older populations they now serve.
2. Developing systems of long-term care.
3. Creating age-friendly environments.
4. Improving measurement, monitoring and understanding.

As previously stated, the main shift towards healthy ageing in 2015 was specifically to address the issue of ageing with health and medical departments or organisations around the world. As a result, three of the four priorities are closely linked to these departments and organisations. Moreover, the two first goals focus on medical care and services in order to foster a geriatric culture in societies which haven't recognised the importance of the challenges of ageing. Taking into account the growing numbers of the ageing population in the immediate future, it can be presumed that this is more than a laudable intention for the WHO.

In contrast, it also delivers a conceptual framework that could emphasise the importance of the environments in the process of ageing which, according to the new definition of healthy ageing, is based on two main concepts: intrinsic capacity and functional ability. Intrinsic capacity is the "combination of individuals and their environments, and the interaction between them" (p. 13) [2]. Functional ability is the central concept of this policy, which states that "Healthy Ageing as the process of developing and maintaining the functional ability that enables well-being in older age" (p. 13) [2].

There are many similarities between the concept of functional ability and that of capability developed by Amartya Sen, the Nobel Prize winner in Economic Sciences in 1998 [4]. This approach is widely accepted in the field of development, even if it is known for its complexity. Roughly, it states that an individual's capabilities are a reflection of the scope of social opportunities or the social context to which they are exposed. The intersection of personal capacities and social opportunities can become capabilities (under certain circumstances). Furthermore, the third objective of the WRAH, "creating age-friendly environments", corresponds exactly to the purpose of proposing different opportunities, by creating a narrative beyond ageism. This social conversation on ageing enhances the adaptation of our built environments that help older adults to live at home longer and within their communities, for as long as they wish or without a social prescription.

17.3 Creating Age-Friendly Cities and Communities (AFCC)

In the following section, we will present the WHO Age-Friendly approach. Firstly, the AFCC approach is a significant achievement of the active ageing framework that was ongoing at the WHO until 2015 [5]. Therefore, it specified that an age-friendly city "… encourages Active Ageing by optimising the health, the participation and the safety of older citizens, in order to improve their quality of life. Concretely, an Age-Friendly City adapts its structures and services so that older persons with diverse capacities and needs can have access to them and take their place within them" (p. 1) [6]. Within the last ten years, there have appeared a multitude of initiatives related to Age-Friendly Cities around the world [7].

The WHO Global Network of Age-Friendly Cities and Communities, established in 2010, now has over 541 members as well as 13 affiliated programmes, in 37 countries, reaching more than 179 million people around the world [8].

Most of these initiatives use a similar model consisting of eight categories where actions can take place which are regularly separated into either built or social environments [9]. The first three categories are outdoor spaces and buildings, transportation and housing. These make up the main core of the built or physical environment. For AFC counsellors this refers to infrastructure, whereas for Public Health Agencies in Canada and Québec, it represents significant social determinants of health. The remaining five categories are: social environment, social participation, respect and inclusion, civic engagement and employment; the last two (communication and information, as well as community support and health services) represent both the social environment and health and social services.

If these categories make sense in the social determinants framework, inherited from the Ottawa Charter, it is difficult to apply them in the daily context of a research [10]. Many countries had to adapt this classification to their realities [7]. However, it gives a broad overview of the areas to tackle in order to ensure that cities and communities are more age-friendly.

The WRAH is now using the *International classification of functioning, disability and health* to upgrade the abilities of a person: "meet basic needs, learn, grow and make decisions, be mobile, build and maintain relationships, to contribute" (p. 19) [2]. If there is no contradiction between this classification and the social determinants framework, then the latter adopts the perspective of the person. For instance, the ability to be mobile is largely conditional to the neighbourhood facilities.

17.4 Defining Age-Friendly Cities or Communities: Québec's Example

Following in the footsteps of the WHO, the Québec government, in Canada, adopted a provincial plan for municipalities to implement the AFCC programme.[1] From its inception in 2008, the government, through the Seniors' Secretariat, which was not

[1] In Québec, this programme is referred to as « Age-Friendly Municipalities » or MADA.

under the jurisdiction of a ministry of health, mandated our research team to lay the foundation of the programme and support seven AFCC projects by ensuring their scientific guidance and support in evaluating the implementation of the proposed projects [11]. Reinforced by the benefits and the knowledge acquired from this research, the programme currently reaches more than 860 municipalities and touches 90% of the Québec population, making it probably one of the most significant AFCC networks in the world.

The AFCC programme consists of three stages carried out over a five-year period and implemented by a steering committee. The role of this committee consists of encouraging commitment and facilitating the realisation of each of the three stages of the AFCC programme, as well as prompting action, circulating information and favouring the mobilisation of actors and decision-makers of the milieu. Unlike an advisory committee, the steering committee plays a much greater role of contribution and collaboration [12]. As well, the sharing of resources (financial, material, human and informational) from different sectors in the milieu often promotes the achievement of common objectives which are more consistent and sustainable. Concretely, the steering committee is a group made up of members of civil society, community workers and leaders of all ages including older adults, originating from various sectors (municipal, public, private, community organisations, etc.).

Based on logic programme approach, the logical sequence of the programme unfolds in three large phases [13]. The first stage of the AFCC programme is the *social diagnosis of the milieu*, in which the municipality does an inventory of its milieu and attempts to generate shared solutions from the actors engaged in the programme. It includes three data-gathering exercises: a statistical portrait of the milieu, an inventory of the services available in the community and discussion groups with older adults to identify their needs. The second stage consists of the *elaboration of an AFCC policy and action plan* corresponding to the gaps and the needs identified during the social diagnosis stage. The action plan is inspired by an approach oriented by a logical framework, as well as on the principles of results-oriented management [14]. It is the members of the steering committee who develop the action plan: its objectives, its inputs, its resources, its activities, its outputs, the persons accountable for it, etc. The final stage, which does not directly benefit from financial support from the AFCC programme, is spread over a period of up to three years. The municipality *implements the AFCC action plan*, carrying out the projects contained in it. The implementation must produce the results anticipated by the action plan and contribute to attaining the objectives set by the steering committee. A financial assistance programme for small infrastructure is open only to municipalities involved in the programme.

17.5 Some Results of the Research

In the first years of the implementation of the programme, the research team conducted cases studies among seven pilot-projects over the course of 5 years. It appeared clearly that one of the keys to success for becoming an Age-Friendly City would be that the different actors should work differently, develop new partnerships, and sometimes the change would entail new governance [15]. For instance, in Québec, health and social services are under the jurisdiction of the provincial ministry of health. Meanwhile the municipal government level is completely separate without any link to the health and social services sector. The experience of the steering committee was often their introduction to working together. We have seen new collaborations blossom to provide better services for older adults. The boldest one is certainly a city project to finance a medical cooperation, which is still in place today.

Moreover, in 2015, a questionnaire was sent by email to 759 municipalities, the total number of participating municipalities between the months of June and September, 2015. They were asked to fill out the electronic version online through the LimeSurvey Internet site (https://www.limesurvey.org/). To ensure the validity and the reliability of the responses, we requested that the questionnaire be completed by one person only, namely the person most closely tied to the AFCC process (e.g. the municipal administrator responsible for the AFCC process, an elected municipal official, a project coordinator). Of the 759 municipalities and Regional County Municipalities (RCMs) solicited, 362 replied to the questionnaire which equates to a response rate of 47.7%. The responding municipalities represent 4,134,531 inhabitants or 49.7% of the Québec population. (A long version of the survey's results is under evaluation for publication.) This undertaking allowed us to obtain much information about the process of the programme: the number of cities which had completed the different steps of the programme (social diagnosis, action plan and implementation), according to size and to the type of programme (e.g. Age-Friendly Cities Programme, or integration with municipal family policy), as well as the level of governance (municipality or RCM). Useful information coming from the survey included: the composition of steering committees, the action fields considered during different stages, the projects they were proud of, etc. We could confirm that (on a large scale) the process allowed municipalities to create new ways of working within their municipal structure. In fact, our data show that 67% of municipalities said they «strongly agree» or «agree» with the fact that the Age-Friendly Cities Programme had allowed them to establish new ways of doing things with the municipal apparatus. With regard to new ways of doing things with their partners, the response rate was 68%.

As we have just seen, the Age-Friendly Cities and Communities model gives interesting results. It encourages a dialogue on ageing between all the different actors who play a role in making environments friendly to older adults. While we need to work on a way to measure progress, the eight active ageing categories make sense for municipalities. It would be unfortunate to abandon them for other referents, some of which may be challenging to individuals, such as the *International classification of functioning, disability and health*. As we often say: why fix what isn't broken?

References

1. Moulaert T, Boudiny K, Paris M (2016) Active and healthy ageing: Blended models and common challenges in supporting age-friendly cities and communities. In: Moulaert T, Garon S (eds) Age-friendly cities and communities in international comparison. Springer, New York, NY, pp 277–304
2. World Health Organization (2015) World report on ageing and health–executive summary. World Health Organization, Geneva. http://who.int/ageing/events/world-report-2015-launch/en/. Accessed 15 Dec 2017
3. Holstein M, Minkler M (2003) Self, society, and the 'new gerontology'. Gerontologist 43:787–796
4. Sen A (1999) Commodities and capabilities. Oxford University Press, New Delhi
5. World Health Organization (2002) Active ageing: a policy framework. World Health Organization, Geneva. http://apps.who.int/iris/bitstream/10665/67215/1/WHO_NMH_NPH_02.8.pdf. Accessed 15 Dec 2017
6. World Health Organization (2007) Global age-friendly cities: a guide. World Health Organization, Geneva. http://www.who.int/kobe_centre/publications/age_friendly_cities_guide/en/. Accessed 15 Dec 2017
7. Moulaert T, Garon S (eds) (2016) Age-friendly cities and communities in international comparison. Springer, New York, NY
8. World Health Organization (2017) Age-friendly world: adding life to years. Website: https://extranet.who.int/agefriendlyworld. Accessed 15 Dec 2017
9. Lui C-W, Everingham J-A, Warburton J, Cuthill M, Bartlett H (2009) What makes a community age-friendly: a review of international literature. Australas J Ageing 28:116–121
10. World Health Organization (1986) Ottawa charter for Health promotion. World Health Organization, Geneva. http://www.who.int/healthpromotion/conferences/previous/ottawa/en/. Accessed 15 Dec 2017
11. Garon S, Veil A, Paris M, Remillard-Boilard S (2016) How can a research program enhance a policy? AFC-Quebec governance and evaluation opportunities. In: Moulaert T, Garon S (eds) Age-friendly cities and communities in international comparison. Springer, New York, NY, pp 99–120
12. Butterfoss FD (2002) Coalitions and partnerships in community health. Wiley, San Francisco
13. Funnell S, Rogers PJ (2011) Purposeful program theory: effective use of theories of change and logics models. Jossey-Bass, San Francisco
14. WK Kellogg Foundation (2004) Evaluation handbook. WK Kellogg Foundation. https://www.bja.gov/evaluation/links/WK-Kellogg-Foundation.pdf. Accessed 15 Dec 2017
15. Garon S, Paris M, Beaulieu M, Veil A, Laliberte A (2014) Collaborative partnership in age-friendly cities: two case studies from Quebec, Canada. J Aging Soc Policy 26:73–87

Healthy Ageing and Health Equity: Broader Determinants of Health with a Spotlight on Climate Change

18

Ritu Sadana, Suman Budhwani, Erik Blas, Ana Posarac, Theadora Koller, and Guillermo Paraje

Key Messages

- Population ageing and climate change are two major drivers of the twenty-first century global context—and warrant experts, civil society and scientific institutions to deliberate and develop plans to optimize healthy ageing and health equity. This will require frameworks that consider common and distinct challenges and entry points for action.
- An appropriate model of healthy ageing therefore requires multi-level determinants and pathways, that can explain the level and distribution of outcomes. We use a social determinants of health model that incorporates biologic approaches; psychosocial approaches; social production of disease distribution; and an

R. Sadana (✉) · A. Posarac
Department of Ageing and Life Course, World Health Organization, Geneva, Switzerland
e-mail: sadanar@who.int

S. Budhwani
Institute of Health Policy, Management and Evaluation, University of Toronto, Toronto, ON, Canada
e-mail: suman.budhwani@mail.utoronto.ca

E. Blas
International Public Health and Development, Copenhagen, Denmark
e-mail: erik@blas.dk

T. Koller
Gender, Equity and Human Rights Team, World Health Organization, Geneva, Switzerland
e-mail: kollert@who.int

G. Paraje
Escuela de Negocios Universidad Adolfo Ibáñez, Santiago, Chile

J.-P. Michel (ed.), *Prevention of Chronic Diseases and Age-Related Disability*, Practical Issues in Geriatrics, https://doi.org/10.1007/978-3-319-96529-1_18

ecological-social framework, and describe three levels of determinants: (1) the physical-socio-economic-political or overall context; (2) genetic inheritance and socioeconomic position; and (3) intermediary determinants including the built environment.

- Climate change is an environmental determinant that can cause unequal health impacts. Older adults can be more vulnerable to the effects of extreme weather events and natural disasters, which can have immediate impacts on mortality and secondary impacts on communicable and noncommunicable diseases.
- Yet there are opportunities to leverage the political momentum of climate change to promote healthy ageing and health equity. Actions that dismantle discrimination, reduce the risk of exposure to and sustained impact from climate change events, improve the adaptive capacity of older adults, and level up socioeconomic conditions, will likely uplift the trajectory of healthy ageing for all people, not just improve conditions for the best-off or the statistical average of all people.

18.1 Introduction

The World Report on Ageing and Health defines *Healthy Ageing* as the process of developing and maintaining the functional ability that enables well-being in older age [1]. Functional ability is "all the health-related attributes that enable people to be and to do what they have reason to value", and is in turn determined by: (1) an individual's intrinsic capacity (i.e. the composite of all the physical and mental capacities of an individual, "within the skin"), (2) the environment (i.e. all the factors in the extrinsic world that form the context of an individual's life) and (3) the interactions between the two. Developing a model of healthy ageing requires a person-centred, dynamic approach, recognizing multilevel determinants and pathways. It should also help explain individual, group, and overall differences, whether within countries or across countries.

Our review of existing evidence on broader determinants of health that are relevant to healthy ageing, points out that much more of the differences in how older adults experience health and illness, not only disease and death, is due to the extent to which an individual, household or group has lived in a society where investments in a safe and healthful environment enable all people over their lives irrespective of their gender, social or economic position, to engage in healthy lifestyles, to enable positive psychosocial interactions, and get effective health and social services based on need and right, rather than pocket book or charity [2]. We agree that when differences exist that can be avoided and are considered unfair, these differences should be labelled as health inequities [3, 4]. *Health equity* implies that ideally everyone should have a fair opportunity to attain their full health potential and that no one should be disadvantaged from achieving this potential.

This chapter primarily discusses social determinants of health model that connects healthy ageing and health equity (drawing on [5]). It also recognizes a nexus of relationships between climate change and social determinants [6], climate change and health inequities [7] and climate change and population ageing [8].

18.2 Towards a Framework for Healthy Ageing and Health Equity

We draw on previous models of ageing [9, 10] and classifications of functioning [11] promoted by WHO and those that have focused on understanding the historical production of inequalities and of health inequities in particular [12–15]. There are several theories reflecting the following four approaches that can be sensibly brought together and inform determinants of healthy ageing: (1) biologic approaches; (2) psychosocial approaches; (3) social production of disease distribution; and (4) eco-social and other multilevel, multi-domain frameworks.

We use the framework developed for the WHO Commission on Social Determinants of Health as a starting point [16]. We also incorporate more recent analyses of this Commission's framework that refine it to describe and explain the health of older adults and the experience of healthy ageing [17–19] as reported in [5]. Recent efforts further extend this across the life course [20, 21] and reiterate the need to go beyond biomedical determinants of the conditions and multiple morbidities older adults experience [22].

Overall, the main pathways and mechanisms through which biologic, social, and environmental factors affect older adults' health are enlightened by several perspectives: (1) biomedical causation (privileging genetic endowment, body functions and medical care); (2) social causation (where social position determines levels of health and its distribution through intermediary factors); (3) life course perspectives (recognizing the importance of time and timing in understanding causal links between exposures and outcomes within an individual's life course, across generations, and in population-level trends in health and survival); and (4) natural environment (includes climate, weather and natural resources such as air, water, soil) as a determinant of human health that recognizes the interaction of all living species and impact on other social determinants of health (includes energy, transport, food, shelter). These approaches are not mutually exclusive, each has merits. Yet alone, none are sufficient to describe the pathways to healthy ageing and respond to the following questions:

1. For older adults, where do health differences across countries and within countries originate, if we trace them back to their deepest roots?
2. What pathways lead from root causes to these stark differences in physical and cognitive functioning and longevity observed at the population level?
3. Where and how should we intervene to reduce health inequities and improve healthy ageing?

It is well documented that genetic, environmental and social influences are important determinants of longevity, health and overall well-being. Hypothesized pathways incorporating risk accumulation, plasticity and resilience models [23] can cut across fundamental, structural, intermediary and proximate determinants, or directly link fundamental environmental factors and cellular impacts [24]. Wallace [18] reviewed evidence on how social determinants affect the health of older adults, and points out the social determinants of health impact ageing and the life course by at least four pathways:

- socioeconomic influences during the prenatal period and early childhood, based on critical periods and events that have direct or indirect latent impacts,
- cumulative health impact of social, economic disadvantage, or privilege,
- sorting people into different life course trajectories, that shape opportunities and chances as they age,
- recognizing intergenerational transmission of health inequities that alter healthy ageing trajectories from birth.

Concerning opportunities to intervene, previous models and frameworks for promoting ageing and health have paid insufficient attention to: political variables; differential impacts and consequences of social and biologic stratification; consideration of sources of resilience or strengths (not only vulnerabilities) that could accumulate over time; and that health and social systems are also intermediary determinants. Some existing models, in particular their policy use, have narrowly summarized ageing as a function of cellular age or declining economic productivity and consumerism, and have concepts and measures limited to static, deficit indicators (e.g. disability, dependency) or noting costs (healthcare expenditures) without the returns on investments.

We conducted a detailed review of all evidence synthesized by the WHO Commission on Social Determinants of Health, including its nine global knowledge networks, from an ageing and health perspective. Even if the Commission did not focus explicitly on ageing and health, life course and cumulative effects of experiences are mentioned throughout. This review also underlined what to highlight in a preliminary model for healthy ageing from an equity and social determinants of health perspective and identify potential policy entry points.

18.2.1 Spotlight on Climate Change

Kjellstrom and McMichael [25] note that any heat, cold, or weather-related reduction of capacity to carry out daily activities that a person values, should be considered a "health effect" and that a variety of direct, indirect, and systemically mediated health effects have been identified, along with additional, future impacts expected given projected climate change. By doing so, they offer a clear connection between climate change and healthy ageing. Although a detailed review of climate change health impacts is beyond the scope of this chapter, in general, warmer temperatures can increase the poleward shift of mosquito-borne diseases (e.g. malaria, dengue, Chikungunya, West Nile) [26] and other vector-borne diseases, such as schistosomiasis and Lyme disease, that can differentially affect specific stages of the life course (e.g. children, pregnant women, older adults), and in different locations (e.g. small island developing states and other coastal regions, megacities, and mountainous and polar regions) [27]. Older adults can be more vulnerable to the effects of extreme weather events and natural disasters, such as flooding, droughts, and wildfires, which can have immediate impacts not only on mortality, but also secondary impacts on communicable and non-communicable disease through increased proneness or exacerbations of existing conditions, for example older adults are at a higher risk of contracting gastrointestinal illnesses from contaminated water [28–32].

Moreover, highly publicized events, such as exceptional heat waves, have increased the risk of death in older populations and have raised the importance of the interaction with other social determinants that exacerbated the risk of death. These include social isolation, and the relative disadvantage of some urban and rural populations who have reduced access to transport, nearby friends, and air-conditioning units [33, 34]. Additional impacts from climate-related adverse events for older adults can include increased probability of disconnect from health and social care supports, inability to adapt as needed during emergencies, and inability to cope following climate-related events [29, 31].

Kjellstrom and McMichael [25] also note that if actions taken to prevent adverse effects of extreme weather conditions inadvertently impair health or well-being, that too should be considered a climate-related "health impact". Thus, understanding the differential impacts that climate change may have on healthy ageing, both intrinsic capacities and functional ability, is part of documenting the accumulation of strengths/resilience or deficits/vulnerabilities across the life course. Yet conversations on healthy ageing do not yet systematically highlight the potential health impacts from climate change on ageing trajectories, nor ways to support integrated risk management, promotion, and adaptation, from a person-centred, equity-enhancing perspective.

But a growing body of literature recognizes the projected impact of climate change on older adults, showcasing their intersection and a particular vulnerability and sensitivity [29–32]. This is both due to demographic and physiological factors often related to ageing processes, and due to factors affecting the degree of exposure to climate stressors, the lived environment and the adaptive capacity of older adults in the face of climate-caused events and circumstances [29, 30, 35]. For example, recent natural disasters due to climate change demonstrated bigger immediate and long-term impacts for older adults than other population groups [31, 36], calling for systematic planning rather than expensive ad hoc, crisis management [37].

18.2.2 Model Components and Policy Entry Points

Figure 18.1 presents a preliminary model with four key components: (1) the physical-socio-economic-political or overall context; (2) genetic inheritance and socioeconomic position; (3) intermediary determinants and (4) the outcome of interest, healthy ageing, including its levels and distributions that take stock of length of life and the experience of healthy ageing.

The healthy ageing framework outlined here starts with the importance attributed to the physical-socio-economic-political context. As Solar and Irwin [16] describe, this is a deliberately broad term that refers to the spectrum of factors in society that cannot be directly measured at the individual level, yet shapes health across the life course and diversity observed across individuals, groups and populations. "Context therefore encompasses a broad set of structural, cultural, natural and functional aspects of a social system whose impact on individuals tends to elude quantification, but which exert a powerful formative influence on patterns of social stratification" and thus on people's health opportunities over the life course. These are also referred to as the "causes of the causes".

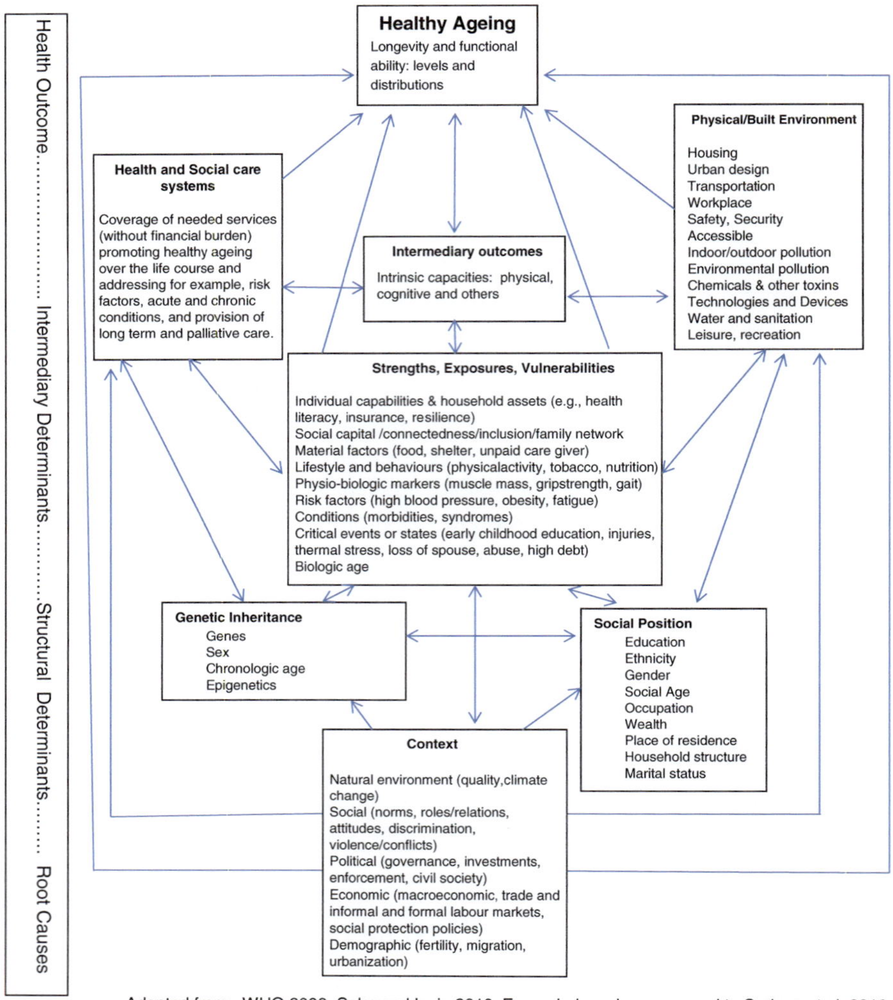

Adapted from: WHO 2008, Solar and Irwin 2010. Expanded version compared to Sadana et al. 2016

Fig. 18.1 Framework for healthy ageing—levels and distribution. Adapted from WHO [2] and Solar and Irwin [16]. Expanded version compared to Sadana et al. [5]

> Almost all of these underlying determinants are amenable to policy change, even though measurable improvements require sustained, coordinated actions. Yet in the context of predictable population ageing, these are very relevant targets for policy actions given the expected returns on investments, and area fundamental if transformational change is to be realized. These policy changes become even more relevant for climate change, which require long-term and short-term actions on multiple policy fronts, to developing concrete strategies to mitigate negative impacts of climate-induced events on older adults [29].

The second block comprises two components influenced by the overall context, that together assign individuals to different positions in society: genetic inheritance and social position. The first, genetic inheritance, is often referred to as "nature":

yet it can reflect biologic intergenerational influences, meaning that genes can be influenced by the environment of our parents, and that the genes individuals inherit can be altered by subsequent environmental exposures and behaviours, both during gestation and once born, over the life course. The second, a significant part of "nurture", is social position, including the social construction of age. Within each society, the degree to which material and other resources, prestige and power are unequally distributed reflects social stratification. The resulting difference in people's lives can be portrayed as a system of social hierarchy and provides insight on how different groups experience healthy ageing and longevity.

> Actions that dismantle discrimination, and level up socioeconomic conditions, will likely uplift the trajectory of healthy ageing for all people. Such actions can theoretically reduce the risk of exposure to and sustained impact from climate change events affecting the health of older adults [29].

The third block shapes the healthy ageing process through intermediary determinants. These include individual level differences in strengths, exposures and vulnerabilities, that reflect social stratification and its interface with genetic inheritance, as well as health-promoting and health-damaging processes and conditions. Reflecting our review of the WHO Commission's evidence, Fig. 18.1 lists key intermediary elements that play an important part in explaining healthy ageing as these link underlying determinants and individual experiences.

As Solar and Irwin [16] describe, these in turn lead to differential consequences of health for more and less advantaged individuals and groups. This bundle of intermediary factors enable or not, the "conversion of resources and primary goods" towards achieving functioning in peoples' lives, and more generally, the ability to achieve what people have reasons to value ([15]: p 33). The intermediary health outcomes are physical, cognitive and other intrinsic capacities, that are person-centred, rather than disease specific.

> In each of the above listed elements, policies at different levels (household, communities, regional, national or global) can improve these determinants and their contribution to realizing healthy ageing. A vast literature exists in this area: the novelty is to place these elements as intermediary determinants, that (a) acknowledges the root causes of the level and distribution of strengths, exposures and vulnerabilities (e.g. that these do not simply reflect individual choice) and (b) considers what are the acute and longer-term opportunities to sustain and increase functional ability through population, community and clinical strategies. For example, relevant to older adults, actions that identify pre-frail and frail individuals, and then support increased physical activity and appropriate nutritional supplements, can potentially reverse frailty and restore physical and cognitive capacities [38].

> Similarly, to reduce or mitigate health impacts from climate change, tools, information and education can be utilized to improve the adaptive capacity of older adults. Adaptation strategies need to address the underlying burden of disease, the interaction within a specific context, and existing inequities. These should address thermal stress, air quality, urban and rural vectors, enteric pathogens, and other health impacts, such as increasing costs of fresh foods, that will more likely affect vulnerable and marginal populations, socioeconomically disadvantaged groups, and those with underlying chronic disease, including older adults [39, 40].

Two sectors or systems are particularly important for improving healthy ageing from an equity perspective. These are also considered as intermediary social determinants: health and social care systems, and the physical or built environment. Each has multiple opportunities to improve healthy ageing, including: (1) crafting policies within each area that promote healthy ageing across the life course, that mediate structural and other intermediary determinants; (2) providing leadership and partnership to other sectors; and (3) as pointed out by the WHO Commission on Social Determinants of Health, mediating the differential consequences of illness in people's lives, where they "live, work, learn and play". This means, for example, to contribute to minimizing the burden of negative consequences that widen the gap between individuals and social groups (e.g. such as regressive financing mechanisms where the poor subsidize the rich; expecting poor families to take care of older family members without support or respite; or in practice serve to exclude the poor from access to needed services). It also means empowering families, care givers and local communities to support older adults where they live, as this is where most older persons want to experience healthy ageing. Context-specific strategies should be developed and discussed with older adults and other stakeholders, to identify and overcome barriers to better adapt to projected climate change [41]. These include adapting and strengthening building codes and urban design, and overall infrastructure capacity.

The final block represents the core outcomes of the healthy ageing process, longevity and optimizing functional ability (intrinsic capacity and interaction with the overall environment). Although preliminary, this framework could be further developed and provide multiple opportunities to better document pathways and policy entry points towards healthy ageing and health equity. Approaches to translate promising entry points to proposals for action are briefly raised in the next section.

18.3 What Could Be Done to Reduce Differences that Are Avoidable, Remediable and Unfair

Building on policy entry points, strategies must not just improve conditions for the best-off or the statistical average of all older persons, but to "level up" the inequalities across the whole social gradient, and to narrow total inequalities observed between individuals. Effective solutions sometimes have to be different approaches for different socioeconomic and demographic groups, otherwise actions could inadvertently increase social stigma, widen inequities and further erode solidarity [42, 43]. Good governance and coordination mechanisms that engage all government and non-governmental sectors, including enabling civil society organizations and older adults themselves to contribute, can support social cohesion, respect decisions reflecting fair processes, catalyse broad based support, and increase accountability [44].

Action to improve healthy ageing and reduce health inequities therefore include (1) action within the health sector or health system including social care and (2) action on the broader social determinants of health—for the latter, these are actions that often lay outside of the health sector or health system. Even if the dividing line between (1) and (2) can vary in each country depending on the boundary of the health sector and health and social systems, multisectoral and intersectoral approaches are essential towards improving health equity. The health sector must take a lead, catalytic role in many areas, and also accept to align and contribute to the goals and actions led by other sectors. For the health system this is crucial, as health programmes generally do not implement interventions that address structural or broader determinants or root causes of inequities.

The impact of climate change and the need for clear action at local level, cities and communities is particularly needed. Urban areas are vulnerable to the health impacts of climate change because of their concentration of people and infrastructure; the physical (geographical, material and structural) attributes of the built environment; and the ecological interdependence with the urban ecosystem [39, 40]. Whereas older adults living in rural areas have long faced significant challenges, with their circumstances shaped by occupations, environments and remoteness [8]. To what extent measures aimed at mitigating climate change serve to reduce or exacerbate health inequities, and to what extent these are complementary or are sources of tension, also need further consideration. For example, reducing carbon emissions, through price mechanisms, could potentially increase income inequality and worsen health inequities [7].

In general, there is evidence that health systems which successfully strive for health equity tend to share several broad features [45–47]. There is also growing evidence for strategies health systems can put in place to support healthy ageing from an equity perspective [48–56]. These include:

- *Catalytic leadership, processes and mechanisms that encourage intersectoral action* across public and private sectors to promote healthy ageing and that cooperate to meet the expectations of these other sectors.
- *Data collection at least by age and sex throughout the life course*, and also by key social characteristics such as income, race, ethnicity, geographic location, among others, that enables the identification of socially patterned differences important for older adults, with total inequalities and social gradients monitored.
- *Strong health system functions, including oversight and governance*: Policies, regulations and incentives in place to ensure that older adults have access to services where ever they live, they age, or social or economic circumstances, without discrimination.
- *Progressive realization of universal (not voluntary) health coverage*, including particular benefits to children and older adults, socially disadvantaged and marginalized groups, and others who are often not adequately covered.
- *Comprehensive approach to understand the broader determinants of healthy ageing*, and the differential exposures and vulnerabilities that individuals and groups may be exposed; and how these approaches can be integrated within care for complex multi-morbidities and long-term care needs.
- *Primary healthcare-centred integrated delivery model for older adults*, which focuses on population-based prevention, health promotion and disease management, with effective coordination between primary, secondary and tertiary

healthcare providers, underpinned by effective financial protection and with links to social care.

- *Health equity concerns incorporated into public health programmes spanning communicable and non-communicable conditions* (such as cardiovascular disease, diabetes, injury prevention and rehabilitation, nutrition, food safety, oral health, mental health, tuberculosis, neglected tropic diseases, alcohol abuse, and tobacco use), as well as for conditions that to date, are often age-dependent (i.e. dementia, stroke, chronic obstructive pulmonary disease; vision, mobility and hearing impairments), for which the burden of disease arises more from experiencing disability and functional decline, than from mortality.
- *Identification and provision of key services* (appropriate, effective, accessible) care across life stages, taking stock that primary prevention in adults aged younger than, for example, 60 years will improve health in successive cohorts of older people; and recognizing that much of the potential to reduce disease burden and improving functional status, will come from more effective primary, secondary, and tertiary prevention.
- *Work force trained, managed and deployed*, with an appropriate skill mix and competences to deliver essential services for older adults, in urban and rural settings.
- *Do not reinforce inequities*, such as discrimination through ageism—in planning, regulations, the way services are delivered, good workforce mix, financing schemes; considers that chronologic age should not be the main criteria to assess health status, nor need for services; addresses signs of elder abuse.
- *Organizational arrangements and practices that involve different population groups*, age groups and civil society organizations that advocate for older adults and "age-friendly" societies more generally—within a fair process and participatory decision-making.

18.4 Next Steps

Currently, all countries have different starting points, yet commitment to take steps and to act for the long term is possible at every level of development. Changes in the age structure of the population, including increases in the proportion of older adults particularly in low and middle income countries, are predictable. There are opportunities to use the political momentum of climate change to promote health equity and healthy ageing. An approach that simultaneously considers factors related to older adults and healthy ageing in conjunction with strategies to mitigate and manage adverse effects of climate change would demonstrate the best results [35]. Even if the projected health impacts of climate change are not pre-determined, where older adults experience social and economic challenges, the exposure and likelihood of health risk due to climate change increases [31].

Recognizing the vulnerability and rights of this population group and enabling the full participation of older adults in developing strategies to mitigate and manage risk from climate-caused events become imperative to ensure reduced health impacts from climate change [31]. Older adults can be mobilized for information due to their historical experiences [31], but also due to their interest in leaving behind a legacy [28, 36]. In addition, optimizing healthy ageing not only includes sufficient preparation of older adults for climate change and its impact, but also developing community capabilities requiring policy implementation at multiple determinant levels [29, 35].

Although all countries could start addressing the health of older adults in a more systematic way now, more evidence describing health inequalities and what can be done that is applicable in diverse contexts is needed that responds to the needs and demands. A WHO global, public consultation to identify important research questions to advance healthy ageing involving more than 1500 respondents in 77 countries during 2016 [57] documented the following important questions spanning research policy, priorities, evidence synthesis and application in communities:

How do we encourage environmental research?

- What environmental factors have most influence on the experience and biology of ageing?
- Can we explore, document and improve climatic conditions, pollution hazards, indoor and outdoor physical infrastructure to render them age-friendly, for better health and well-being?
- What can be done about strengthening environments against extreme environmental events/disasters (in general but also as they relate to older adults), as e.g. a massive solar flare shutting down the electrical grid?
- What type of housing could be proposed for older persons in a world subjected to climatic change?
- What are the effects of climate change on design of age-friendly environments? How can climate change affect initiatives to create an age-friendly environment, in the setting of Small Islands development states?
- How can we build community resilience to changing climate and environment?
- How can we provide older adults accurate information on how their environment impacts their health so they can make useful decisions?
- What role can design and technology play in making outdoor environments more accessible and age-friendly?
- Can a dynamic indicator for healthy ageing be constructed, not absolute but relativized to climate conditions, social context, and ways of communication?

Hudson aptly notes that "If much aging-related research and practice is based on what has gone before, climate change and its challenges— affecting people of all ages and those yet to be born—has a distinct forward thrust" [36]. Population ageing and climate change reflect this century's challenges, and warrant experts, civil society and scientific institutions to deliberate and develop plans. This process would contribute to developing a research and action agenda from an equity perspective, that fully embraces a wide spectrum of environmental and social determinants of healthy ageing. Documenting what is being done at local levels, such as through WHO's Global Network for Age-friendly Cities and Communities, would offer an important source of practice.

On the other, actions can already be taken by governments to enable a comprehensive response more generally [44], that increases alignment between existing policy commitments [58], and adequate resources to "level up" societies in terms of opportunities for health. This is the case given the political mandate of WHO Member States to implement the WHO Global Strategy on Ageing and Health [59].

We aimed to connect healthy ageing and health equity, by raising awareness of inequalities, determinants, and what could be done to improve health equity. We note underlying and intermediate causes of inequities in healthy ageing and review existing evidence on what could be done to improve healthy ageing from an equity perspective. Using this model, we highlight the importance of climate change, impacts on older adults, and the need to further knowledge and evidence based actions connecting climate change and healthy ageing.

Acknowledgments This chapter draws on a background paper [4] prepared for the *WHO World Report on Ageing and Health* and adds new material on climate change reflecting a WHO Global public consultation on research priorities for healthy ageing, supported by The Velux Stiftung.

Disclaimer: RS and TK are staff members of the World Health Organization. All listed authors alone are responsible for the views expressed in this publication and they do not necessarily represent the decisions, policy or views of the World Health Organization.

References

1. World Health Organization (2015) World report on ageing and health. WHO, Geneva
2. WHO (2008) Commission on social determinants of health final report. World Health Organization, Geneva. http://www.who.int/social_determinants/thecommission/finalreport/en/index.html
3. Braveman P, Gruskin S (2003) Defining equity in health. J Epidemiol Community Health 57:254–259
4. Whitehead M (1992) The concepts and principles of equity and health. Int J Health Ser 22:429–445
5. Sadana R, Blas E, Budhwani S, Koller T, Paraje G (2016) Healthy ageing: raising awareness of inequalities, determinants, and what can be done to improve health equity. Gerontologist 56(2):S178–S193
6. Friel S, Marmot M, McMichael A, Kjellstrom T, Vågerö D (2008) Global health equity and climate stabilisation: a common agenda. Lancet 372:1677–1683. PMID: 18994666. https://doi.org/10.1016/S0140-6736(08)61692-X
7. Walpole SC, Rasanathan K, Campbell-Lendrum D (2009) Natural and unnatural synergies: climate change policy and health equity. Bull World Health Organ 87:799–801. https://doi.org/10.2471/BLT.09.067116
8. Horton G, Hanna L, Kelly B (2010) Drought, drying and climate change: emerging health issues for ageing Australians in rural areas. Australas J Ageing 29:2–7. https://doi.org/10.1111/j.1741-6612.2010.00424.x
9. Kuh D, Cooper R, Hardy R, Richards M, Ben-Shlomo Y (eds) (2014) A life course approach to healthy ageing. Oxford University Press, Oxford
10. WHO (2002) Active ageing policy framework. WHO, Geneva. WHO/NMH/NPH/028
11. WHO (2001) International classification of functioning, disability and health (ICF). World Health Organization, Geneva

12. Davey Smith G (2003) In: Davey Smith G (ed) Health inequalities: life course approaches. The Policy Press, London
13. Diderichsen F (1998) Understanding health equity in populations. In: Avre-Pares B (ed) Promoting research on inequality in health. Swedish Council for Social Research, Stockholm, pp 99–114
14. Krieger N (2014) Got theory?—on the 21st century rise of explicit use of epidemiologic theories of disease distribution: a review and ecosocial analysis. Curr Epidemiol Rep 1:45–56. https://doi.org/10.1007/s40471-013-0001-1
15. Sen A (1992) Inequality reexamined. Russell Sage Foundation, Harvard University Press, New York, Cambridge
16. Solar O, Irwin A (2010) World Health Organization: a conceptual framework for action on the social determinants of health. Social determinants of health discussion paper 2 (policy and practice). http://www.who.int/social_determinants/publications/9789241500852/en/
17. Sadana R, Foebel AD, Williams AN, Beard JR (2013) Population ageing, longevity, and the diverse contexts of the oldest old. Public Policy Aging Rep 23(2):18–25
18. Wallace (2012) Social determinants of health inequities and health care in older age. In: Prohaska TR, Anderson LA, Binstock RH (eds) Public health for an aging Soceity. Johns Hopkins University Press, Baltimore, MD
19. Zaidi A (2014) Life cycle transitions and vulnerabilities in old age: a review. UNDP Human Development Report Office Occasional Paper. http://hdr.undp.org/sites/default/files/hdr_2014_zaidi_final.pdf
20. Bell R, Marmot M (2017) Life course approach to understanding inequalities in health in later life. In: Michel JP, Beattie BL, Martin FC, Walston JD (eds) Oxford textbook of geriatric medicine, 3rd edn. Oxford University Press, Oxford. https://doi.org/10.1093/med/9780198701590.003.0010
21. Kuruvilla S, Sadana R, Villar Montesinos E et al (2018) A life-course approach to health: synergy with sustainable development goals. Bull World Health Organ 96:42–50
22. Northwood M, Ploeg J, Markle-Reid M, Sherifali D. Integrative review of the social determinants of health in older adults with multimorbidity. J Adv Nurs 2018;74:45–60. 10.1111/jan.13408
23. Kuh D, Ben-Shlomo Y, Lynch J et al (2003) Life course epidemiology. J Epidemiol Community Health 57:778–783
24. Adams JM, White M (2004) Biological ageing: a fundamental, biological link between socio-economic status and health? Eur J Pub Health 14(3):331–334
25. Kjellstrom T, McMichael AJ (2013) Climate change threats to population health and well-being: the imperative of protective solutions that will last. Glob Health Action 6:20816. https://doi.org/10.3402/gha.v6i0.20816
26. Servadio JL, Rosenthal SR, Carlson L, Bauer C (2018) Climate patterns and mosquito-borne disease outbreaks in south and Southeast Asia. J Infect Public Health 11(4):566–571. https://doi.org/10.1016/j.jiph.2017.12.006
27. WHO (2012) Ten facts on climate change and health. World Health Organization. http://www-whoint/features/factfiles/climate_change/en/. Accessed 27 Feb 2018
28. Frumkin H, Fried L, Moody R (2012) Aging, climate change, and legacy thinking. Am J Public Health 102(8):1434–1438
29. Gamble JL, Hurley BJ, Schultz PA, Jaglom WS, Krishnan N, Harris M (2013) Climate change and older Americans: state of the science. Environ Health Perspect 121(1):15–22
30. Gamble JL, Balbus J, Berger M, Bouye K, Campbell V, Chief K, Conlon K, Crimmins A, Flanagan B, Gonzalez-Maddux C, Hallisey E, Hutchins S, Jantarasami L, Khoury S, Kiefer M, Kolling J, Lynn K, Manangan A, McDonald M, Morello-Frosch R, Redsteer MH, Sheffield P, Thigpen Tart K, Watson J, Whyte KP, Wolkin AF (2016) Ch. 9. Populations of concern. The impacts of climate change on human health in the United States: a scientific assessment. U.S. Global Change Research Program, Washington, DC, pp 247–286. https://doi.org/10.7930/J0Q81B0T

31. HelpAge (2016) Climate change in an ageing world: HelpAge position paper. HelpAge International, London
32. United States Environmental Protection Agency (2016) Climate change and the health of older adults. https://archive.epa.gov/epa/sites/production/files/2016-10/documents/older-adults-health-climate-change.pdf
33. Davido A, Patzak A, Dart T et al (2006) Risk factors for heat related death during the August 2003 heat wave in Paris, France, in patients evaluated at the emergency department of the Hopital Europeen Georges Pompidou. Emerg Med J 23:515–518
34. Semenza JC, Rubin CH, Falter KH et al (1996) Heat-related deaths during the July 1995 heat wave in Chicago. N Engl J Med 335:84–90
35. Institute for Science (2018) Innovation and Society. University of Oxford http://www.future-ofcities.ox.ac.uk/research/climate-change-and-the-ageing-population/
36. Hudson RB (2017) Gray and green together: climate change in an aging world. Public Policy Aging Rep 27(1):1–3. https://doi.org/10.1093/ppar/prw051
37. Burton AJ, Bambrick HJ, Friel S (2014) Is enough attention given to climate change in health service planning? An Australian perspective. Glob Health Action 7(1):23903. https://doi.org/10.3402/gha.v7.23903
38. Michel JP, Cruz-Jentoft AJ, Cederholm T (2015) Frailty, exercise and nutrition. Clin Geriatr Med 31(3):375–387
39. Bambrick H, Dear K, Woodruff R, Hanigan I, McMichael A. (2008) The impacts of climate change on three health outcomes: temperature-related mortality and hospitalisations, salmonellosis and other bacterial gastroenteritis, and population at risk from dengue. Garnaut Climate Change Review. http://garnautreview.org.au/CA25734E0016A131/WebObj/03-AThreehealthoutcomes/$File/03-A%20Three%20health%20outcomes.pdf. Accessed 29 Dec 2017
40. Brambrick H, Capon AG, Barnett GB et al (2011) Climate change and health in the urban environment: adaptation opportunities in Australian cities. Asia Pac J Public Health 23(2 Suppl):67S–79S
41. Zhang Y, Wang JN, Ma W, Nitschke M, Hansen A, Bi P, Jiang BF (2016) Case study: improving population health in a rapidly urbanizing world: are older Chinese people ready to adapt to climate change? In: Urbanization and public health in China, pp 267–298. https://doi.org/10.1142/9781783268559_0013
42. Popay J et al (2008) Understanding and tackling social exclusion. (Final report of the social exclusion knowledge network of the commission on social determinants of health). World Health Organization, Geneva
43. Wood R, Sutton M, Clark D, McKeon A, Bain M (2006) Measuring inequalities in health: the case for healthy life expectancy. J Epidemiol Community Health 60:1089–1092. https://doi.org/10.1136/jech.2005.044941
44. Blas E, Gilson L, Kelly MP et al (2008) Addressing social determinants of health inequities: what can the state and civil society do? Lancet 372:1684–1689
45. Blas E, Sivasankara-Kurup A (eds) (2010) Equity, social determinants of health and public health programmes. World Health Organization, Geneva http://apps.who.int/iris/bitstream/10665/44289/1/9789241563970_eng.pdf
46. Gilson L, Doherty J, Loewenson R, Francis V et al (2007) Challenging inequity through health systems. (Final report of the health systems knowledge network of the commission on social determinants of health). World Health Organization, Geneva http://www.who.int/social_determinants/resources/csdh_media/hskn_final_2007_en.pdf
47. Sadana R, Blas E (2013) What can public health programs do to improve health equity? Public Health Rep 128(Suppl 3):12–20
48. Bloom ED, Mahal A, Rosenberge L (2012) Design and operation of health systems in developing countries. Global population ageing: peril or promise? Global Agenda Council on Ageing Society, World Economic Forum
49. HelpAge (2013) Global AgeWatch index 2013: insight report. HelpAge International, London

50. HelpAge (2014) Global AgeWatch index 2014: insight report. HelpAge International, London
51. HelpAge (2015) Global AgeWatch index 2015: insight report. HelpAge International, London
52. Marmot M (2012) Review of social determinants and the health divide in the WHO European region. World Health Organization, Regional Office for Europe, Copenhagen
53. Prince MJ, Wu F, Guo Y et al (2015) The burden of disease in older people and implications for health policy and practice. Lancet 385(9967):549–562. https://doi.org/10.1016/S0140-6736(14)61347-7
54. Yip W, Hsiao W (2014) Harnessing the privatisation of China's fragmented health-care delivery. Lancet 384(9945):805–818
55. WHO (2010) The world health report 2010–the path to financing universal health coverage. World Health Organization, Geneva
56. WHO (2014) Making fair choices on the path to universal health coverage. Final report of the WHO consultative group on equity and universal health coverage. WHO, Geneva. http://www.who.int/choice/documents/making_fair_choices/en/
57. WHO (2018) Building research policy on health ageing: evidence gaps, public consultation and strategic engagement. WHO series on metrics, research and knowledge translation, paper 3. World Health Organization, Geneva
58. Baker P, Friel S, Kay A, Baum F, Strazdins L, Mackean T (2018) What enables and constrains the inclusion of the social determinants of health inequities in government policy agendas? A narrative review. Int J Health Policy Manag 7(2):101–111. https://doi.org/10.15171/ijhpm.2017.130
59. World Health Organization (2017) WHO global strategy and action plan on ageing and health. WHO, Geneva

Integrated Care for Older People

19

Islène Araujo de Carvalho, Joanne Epping-Jordan, and John R. Beard

Key Messages

- To face the increasing demands of healthcare by the growing number of older adults, segmented care system has to be replaced by person-centred and integrated care.
- This includes a comprehensive assessment able to identify health and social care needs of older people.
- The responses to these increased demands include supportive policies, plans and regulatory frameworks.
- Indeed I-technology communication will help increasing training of healthcare workers to provide personalized care to allow older persons to do what matter for them until the latest part of life.
- Actions towards delivery of integrated care for the older people can take place at all levels of healthcare.

19.1 The Policy Context

19.1.1 Rapid Demographic Changes

At a time of unpredictable public health challenges, one thing is certain: the world's population is rapidly ageing. From 2015 to 2050, the proportion of the world's population aged 60 years or older will nearly double (from 12 to 22%) [1]. The consequences for healthcare systems are profound.

I. A. de Carvalho (✉) · J. R. Beard
WHO, Department of Ageing and Life Course, Geneva Headquarters, Geneva, Switzerland
e-mail: araujodecarvalho@who.int

J. Epping-Jordan
Seattle, WA, USA

J.-P. Michel (ed.), *Prevention of Chronic Diseases and Age-Related Disability*, Practical Issues in Geriatrics, https://doi.org/10.1007/978-3-319-96529-1_19

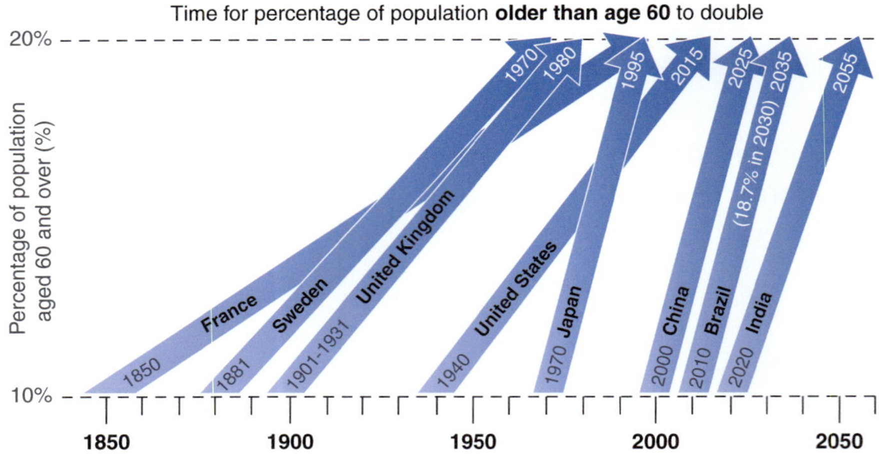

Fig. 19.1 Pace of demographic transition. Source: WHO World Report on Ageing and Health, 2015

As depicted in the Fig. 19.1 below, the rate at which the proportion of the population aged ≥60 years is increasing much more quickly than in the past [1]. For example, the proportion of the French population that was older than 60 years rose from 10 to 20% over a period of almost 150 years, whereas countries such as China and India will have only slightly more than 20 years to adjust to similar changes in the age structure of their populations. A child born in Brazil or Myanmar in 2015 can expect to live 20 years longer than one born just 50 years ago [1].

19.1.2 Diverse Healthcare Needs

As people age, their *intrinsic capacity*—the sum of their physical and mental capacities—tends to decline while their health issues become more chronic and complex. Multimorbidity—the presence of multiple chronic conditions at the same time—is increasingly prevalent with age. Older people can develop geriatric syndromes such as frailty, urinary incontinence, and falls, which do not fall into discrete disease categories.

19.1.3 Challenges and Complexities in Providing Healthcare to Older Populations

Health systems around the world are struggling to respond to the wide diversity of physical and mental capacities of older people and to promote positive trajectories of healthy ageing from early life onwards. An older person's capacities can change rapidly—over the course of hours in some cases. Care systems struggle to be nimble enough to respond quickly to alterations in a person's needs.

Numerous healthcare workers may be involved with one person's care, especially in countries with extensive availability of medical specialists.

The social care sector is often involved when older people experience significant declines in their capacities and need help with activities of daily living. Health and social care services for older people are typically provided in a range of diverse settings, and with greater frequency, than for younger populations. In addition, families and other unpaid carers often play substantial caregiving roles [2].

19.1.4 Healthcare Mismatch

Many healthcare systems around the world were designed for a relatively young population and for a different set of health needs than those we face today. In the past, services were often structured to diagnose and cure acute health issues, using a biomedical 'find it and fix it' approach, which worked well when communicable diseases were the most prevalent healthcare issue. Even though population demographics have shifted, the clinical focus often remains on the detection and treatment of acute conditions, while attention to problems that matter to older people—such as chronic pain, and management of ongoing difficulties with hearing, seeing, walking or performing daily activities—tends to be overlooked. Protocols are often lacking for preventing and managing geriatric issues such as frailty and urinary incontinence. Early markers of declines in intrinsic capacity, such as decreases in gait speed or muscle strength, are often not identified, treated or monitored, which is crucial if they are to be reversed or delayed.

Older people's health issues also are often managed in disconnected and fragmented ways, and there is little coordination between care providers, different settings and over time. Yet, the involvement of numerous health professionals and the use of multiple clinical interventions necessitate a high degree of coordination, both between health professionals, and within treatment levels and settings.

The physical infrastructure of many healthcare settings is not well matched to older people's needs. This includes a lack of accessible toilets, long waiting lines, physical barriers to access, and communication barriers resulting from a lack of accessible information for people with hearing loss and visual impairment. The shortage of affordable transportation to clinics is another major barrier to accessing healthcare, especially for older people who live in rural areas, because services are often concentrated in large cities far from older people's homes and communities [3].

Finally, healthcare and social care are typically fragmented from one another. Deeply rooted differences in the way that these services are financed, governed, and organized create complications for older people who use both types of services. Separate budgets and competing incentives for the various organizations are not conductive to care coordination. Differences in education and professional culture, and unfamiliarity with other professionals' ways of working, are additional barriers.

19.1.5 Poorly Prepared Healthcare Workers

Like healthcare systems, healthcare workers are often unprepared to effectively manage the healthcare needs of older adults. Most current training approaches were developed in the twentieth century [4], when acute, communicable conditions were the world's most prevalent health problems. As a result, healthcare workers are often trained to respond to pressing health concerns, rather than to proactively anticipate and counteract changes in function; and they are rarely prepared to work with older people to ensure they can increase control over their own health [4–6]. Furthermore, although most patients treated within health systems are older people, training curricula frequently overlook gerontological and geriatric knowledge and training [7, 8] and may lack guidance on the management of common problems such as multimorbidity and frailty.

Meaningful reform will require the concerted and sustained efforts of academic leaders and health professional groups, but, so far, this has not happened to a large degree.

19.2 Responses

19.2.1 Integrated Care for Older People

Evidence suggests that *integrated care for older people* is the best approach for implementing the complex spectrum of interventions that are needed for older people to experience the best possible outcomes [9–12].

Integrated care for older people refers to services that span the care continuum; are integrated within and among the different levels and sites of care within the healthcare and long-term care systems (including within the home); and according to people's needs throughout the life course. Integration does not mean that structures must merge, but rather, that a wide array of service providers must work together in a coordinated way. Experiences to date [13, 14] indicate that most successful programmes have taken a bottom-up approach to change, which has been supported by higher-level policy and mechanisms for shared financing and accountability within teams.

This type of care is person-centred, which means that it is grounded in the perspective that older people are more than vessels of their disorders or health conditions. Instead, they are viewed as individuals with unique experiences, needs, and preferences. They also are seen in the context of their daily lives, as part of a family and a community.

To illustrate the elements of this type of care, WHO proposed in the 2015 WHO World Report on Ageing and Health actions in three levels (below). Key actions at three levels:

1. *Focus on the older person's needs and goals.* All elements of an integrate care approach for older people revolve around each older person's unique needs and goals.

2. *Integrated clinical care.* Integration at the level of clinical care is especially important for older populations. This includes a comprehensive assessment, a common goal, and a care plan that is shared across all providers.
3. *System alignment.* Aligned health and long term care systems can enable the realization of integrated care for older people. Key building blocks of health systems have been identified previously by WHO [15] and include: Service delivery; human resources for health; health infrastructure, products, vaccines and technologies; information and data, leadership and governance, and financing.

19.2.2 What Can Healthcare Providers Do?

Front-line health workers who deliver care to older people can take several steps to provide more integrated care to older people. These include: using case management strategies, including comprehensive assessments, care plans, and proactive follow-up; implementing evidence-based clinical interventions tailored to level of intrinsic capacity; and working collaboratively with other providers.

1. *Undertake case management.* Case management entails assessing individual needs and developing a comprehensive care plan (see below), and then organizing services so they work collectively towards the goal of maintaining intrinsic capacity [16].
   (a) *Conduct comprehensive assessments.* Comprehensive assessments are an essential aspect of case management. They take stock of the intrinsic capacity of the older person and its trajectory; specific conditions, behaviours, and risks that may influence this in the future; and the environmental context. As such, comprehensive assessments provide the information needed to prioritize and tailor interventions.
   - *Set care goals together with the older person.* It is crucial that the older person is involved with decision-making and goal setting from the outset, and that goals are established in accordance with the older person's unique needs and preferences.

   (b) *Develop and use comprehesive care plans.* These are developed based on the outcomes of comprehensive assessments. The care plan is centred around the older person's goals, how they will be addressed, the roles that different sectors of the health and social system will play, and a plan for follow-up and re-assessment. Once the care plan is developed, it serves as a roadmap for unified action and a way of measuring progress against the older person's individual goals and preferences.
   - *Provide systematic self-management support.* This involves providing older people with the information, skills, and tools that they need to manage their health conditions, prevent complications, maximize their intrinsic capacity, and maintain their quality of life [17, 18]. This does not imply that older people will be expected to 'go it alone' or that unreasonable or excessive demands will be placed on them. It does, however, recognize their autonomy

and abilities to direct their own care, in consultation and partnership with healthcare providers, their families and a range of other carers.

- *Provide regular and sustained follow-up.* Proactive and planned follow-up is part of most case management approaches. It promotes early detection of complications or changes in functional status, thus preventing unnecessary emergencies and related healthcare waste. It also provides a forum to monitor progress in relation to the care plan and to provide additional support as needed.

(c) *Implement evidence-based clinical interventions tailored to levels of intrinsic capacity.* Within any population of older people, many will experience periods of high and stable capacity, declining capacity, and significant loss of capacity. Each of these three periods requires different responses from healthcare providers.

- *For older people with high and stable levels of capacity, the goal is to build and maintain these levels for as long as possible.* The emphasis should be on disease and risk prevention; promoting capacity-enhancing behaviours; ensuring acute problems are adequately addressed; and detecting and managing chronic, noncommunicable diseases at an early stage.
- *For older people experiencing declining capacity, the goal is to delay, slow, or even partly reverse this trajectory through interventions targeted early in the process* [19, 20]. Healthy behaviours remain crucial, but the focus broadens from risk factor reduction to encompass actions that can directly help maintain and reverse loss in intrinsic capacity. For example, aerobic exercise is important for cardiovascular disease prevention [21], but exercise that can help build muscle mass, strength, and balance becomes increasingly important as people begin to experience declining capacity [22–27]. Nutritional advice also changes as people lose capacity, with the focus shifting to nutrient density, particularly that of protein intake, vitamin D, and other micronutrients, although calorie intake is also an important target [28]. This is a period of increased focus on the chronic care of multiple conditions, in order to mitigate their impact on capacity.
- *For older people experiencing significant loss of capacity, the twin goals are to continue to optimize clinical trajectories and to compensate for these losses through provision of social care services.* Clinical interventions should continue to focus on recovering and maintaining capacity, including ongoing disease management, rehabilitation, palliative interventions, and end of life care. Rehabilitation services can help prevent permanent functional disability and care dependency, and have been shown to reduce avoidable hospital admissions and delayed discharges [29].

2. *Work collaboratively with other providers.* Integrated care for older people requires healthcare providers to collaborate with one another, and with social care providers. This is a different way of working for many providers. Differences in education and professional culture, and unfamiliarity with other professionals' ways of working must be overcome.

19.2.3 How Can Services Be Organized and Delivered?

The starting point for aligning services to support integrated care for older people should be ensuring that better care is provided, rather than adopting a fixed organizational model with a pre-determined design.

Regardless of the organizational structure, active case finding, community- and home-based care—all anchored by a strong and high-performing primary health and long term care system—are important aspects of service delivery for older people. Self-management support provides older people with the information, skills, and tools that they need to manage their health conditions; prevent complications; maximize their intrinsic capacity; and maintain their quality of life. Community engagement leverages existing resources and helps provide support for older people and their families.

1. *Use multidisciplinary teams*. Multidisciplinary teams share responsibility and accountability for clinical processes and care outcomes, for individuals and in defined populations. To succeed, teams meet regularly, share information, explicitly define clinical roles, and perform complementary and coordinated functions for people and populations [30].
2. *Share information across providers, settings, and time*. Rapid advances in information and communication technologies (ICTs) offer much promise for sharing relevant clinical information across providers, settings, and time [31]. Electronic health records can organize information about individuals and entire clinical populations of older people to help identify needs, plan care over time, monitor responses to treatment, and assess health outcomes.
   (a) *Implement active case finding*. Community outreach and active case finding can reach older people who do not self-present to health centres. Moving beyond clinic walls into communities facilitates the identification, monitoring, and support of older people in need of health services.
3. *Prioritize community- and home-based care*. Locating health services close to where people live is especially important for older people. Distances to health centres that might be reasonable for the general population can be insurmountable for older people with significant impairments; accessible and affordable public transportation to healthcare facilities should be available [32]. In cases where specialist health services entail long travel distances, age-friendly and affordable transportation services can be offered.

   Home visits delivered by healthcare providers in the context of community-based programmes have been shown to have positive effects for older people [33, 34].

   For those with significant care needs, hospital-at-home services can provide treatment at home for people who would otherwise be admitted to an acute hospital. These services involve a team of health and long-term care professionals. Evidence has shown higher client and carer satisfaction, reduced deaths, and reduced readmission rates with this model compared to a 'traditional' hospital [35]. Most rehabilitation services can be provided outside hospital settings, in communities or at home [28].

(a) *Engage communities*. Community engagement leverages untapped resources and helps to ensure healthy and facilitative environments for older people. The community includes families and households, employers, religious organizations, the physical and social environment, community organizations of different types—including older people's associations, social services, and educational services to name but a few.

19.2.4 How Can Health and Long Term Care Systems Support Integrated Care?

The primary role for policymakers and health system leaders is to support the integration activities of front-line providers at the level of clinical care (see Box below).

National-Level Support for Integrated Care for Older People

1. Adopt an integrated care approach to older people within the country's National Health Policy.
2. Adapt and implement clinical guidelines for providing integrated care for older people.
3. Evaluate the country's capacity to deliver integrated care, identify gaps, develop a plan, and monitor progress.
4. Make needed changes within local health systems (essential medicines, health information system, infrastructure) and long term care systems.
5. Train health and social workers about the integrated care approach and interventions to prevent declines in capacity and functional abilities.
6. Develop support mechanisms within communities for self-management, caregiver support, and transportation of older people to clinics and hospitals when needed.

Organizational and structural integration are not necessary to achieve this aim.

As a first step, senior leaders must recognize the importance of addressing this agenda and make it a health system priority. One entry point is to evaluate the country's capacity to deliver integrated care, identify gaps, elaborate a plan to guide the necessary changes in local health systems, and monitor progress.

Policies, plans, and regulatory frameworks can be updated to support integration at care levels (e.g. primary healthcare, nursing homes, and hospital-based services), and also between health and long term care systems. Joint budgeting, monitoring, and accountability systems can be used to solidify integration. Strong political support from senior leadership can spur this type of action.

Other essential action points are presented below.

1. *Develop the workforce*. Healthcare and social care workers need the right competencies, and to be organized and deployed in ways that make the best

use of their potential contributions. Core competencies for all health professionals include basic gerontological and geriatric skills. Both health and social care workers need general competencies related to integrated care, such as working as part of a multidisciplinary team and proactively supporting older people to optimize their health and capacity. More physicians and nurses with expertise in geriatrics are also needed, to provide support to primary care healthcare workers and to treat complex cases. In addition, new workforce cadres (such as care coordinators or community health workers) can be considered, alongside options for extending the permissible scope of practice for some professions.

Developing the workforce in these ways will require a well-functioning governance infrastructure. Workforce assessment, policy development, planning and monitoring are essential aspects of governance. Strengthening governance capacities and coordination mechanisms to address major workforce challenges associated with population ageing will be important in many settings.

(a) *Invest in information and communication technologies.* Information and communication technologies (ICT) can help transform health systems to deliver integrated care for older people, particularly in middle- and high-income settings. Advances in ICT are being used globally to improve access, quality, and safety of healthcare, and cost-effectiveness of health services delivery [30]. In many ways, ICT has become fundamental to effective multidisciplinary team care. Automated reminders, prompts, and warnings on clinical health records systems can assist providers to deliver evidence-based care. Patient portals and other e-health infrastructure can enable older people to participate more fully in their treatment and care; and link them with their healthcare team, as well as with community and social services.

    ICT also can be used to monitor, evaluate, and plan care at the policy level, in order to improve the care of older people. For this to be realized, common indicators must be broadly agreed and consistently used. Indicators for underlying causes and domains of intrinsic capacity—such as undernutrition, mobility impairment, cognitive impairment, and sensory impairments—must be defined, operationalized, and consistently measured.

2. *Implement shared financing and accountability.* Several financing mechanisms can be considered to stimulate integrated care for older people. Within a wide range of financing schemes, pooled budgets and/or bundled payments can be used to enable providers and organizations to work together in a more integrated way. Other financing mechanisms include contractual incentives to encourage new ways of working, or to reward positive outcomes; and stimulus or seed funding to support the development of local initiatives.

   Regardless of the financing scheme, providers must be compensated and provided with incentives to undertake key functions associated with integrated care. They must, for example, be remunerated for the time and resources spent conducting comprehensive assessments and developing care plans, as well as for the time spent on consultation and collaboration within the multidisciplinary team. Providers should also be eligible for compensation related to the services that they provide in older people's homes or communities.

Conclusion

Integrated care for older people produces a better return on investment than more familiar ways of working, and enables older people to participate and contribute as productive members of society [1].

Integration at the level of clinical care is especially important for older populations. This generally includes a comprehensive assessment, a common goal, and a care plan that is shared across all providers. Ongoing case management, led by a designated care coordinator, has been shown to ensure that integration continues over time [2]. Key health system levers are: supportive policies, plans, and regulatory frameworks; workforce development; investment in information and communication technologies; and use of pooled budgets, bundled payments, and contractual incentives to support integrated ways of working.

Action towards the delivery of integrated care for older people can take place at all levels of healthcare: from front-line providers through to senior leaders. This action might make a substantial contribution towards the Sustainable Development Goals (SDGs), fostering inclusive economic growth, achieving universal health coverage for current and future populations, and ensuring older people have the opportunity to contribute to—and are not left behind by—development.

References

1. WHO (2015) World report on ageing and health. World Health Organization, Geneva
2. Osborn R, Moulds D, Squires D et al (2014) International survey of older adults finds shortcomings in access, coordination, and patient-centered care. Health Aff (Millwood) 33:2247–2255
3. Balarajan Y, Selvaraj S, Subramanian SV (2011) Health care and equity in India. Lancet 377:505–515
4. Frenk J, Chen L, Bhutta ZA et al (2010) Health professionals for a new century: transforming education to strengthen health systems in an interdependent world. Lancet 376:1923–1958
5. Pruitt SD, Epping-Jordan JE (2005) Preparing the 21st century global healthcare workforce. BMJ 330:637–639
6. Institute of Medicine (2008) Retooling for an aging America: building the health care workforce. The National Academies Press, Washington, DC
7. Mateos-Nozal J, Beard JR (2011) Global approaches to geriatrics in medical education. Eur Geriatr Med 2:87–92
8. WHO (2002) Global survey on geriatrics in the medical curriculum. World Health Organization, Geneva
9. McDonald KM, Schultz EM, Chang C (2013) Evaluating the state of quality-improvement science through evidence synthesis: insights from the closing the quality gap series. Perm J 17:52–61
10. Ouwens M, Wollersheim H, Hermens R et al (2005) Integrated care programmes for chronically ill patients: a review of systematic reviews. Int J Qual Health Care 17:141–146
11. Nolte E, Pitchforth E (2014) What is the evidence on the economic impacts of integrated care? Policy summary 11. World Health Organization, Geneva
12. Johri M, Beland F, Bergman H (2003) International experiments in integrated care for the elderly: a synthesis of the evidence. Int J Geriatr Psychiatry 18:222–235
13. Wodchis WP, Dixon A, Anderson GM et al (2015) Integrating care for older people with complex needs: key insights and lessons from a seven-country cross-case analysis. Int J Integr Care 15:e021

14. Goodwin N, Dixon A, Anderson GM et al (2014) Providing integrated care for older people with complex needs: lessons from seven international case studies. The King's Fund, London
15. WHO (2007) Everybody's business: strengthening health systems to improve health outcomes: WHO's framework for action. World Health Organization, Geneva
16. Goodwin N, Sonola L, Thiel V et al (2013) Co-ordinated care for people with complex chronic conditions. The King's Fund, London
17. Nunez DE, Keller C, Ananian CD (2009) A review of the efficacy of the self-management model on health outcomes in community-residing older adults with arthritis. Worldviews Evid-Based Nurs 6:130–148
18. Sherifali D, Bai JW, Kenny M et al (2015) Diabetes self-management programmes in older adults: a systematic review and meta-analysis. Diabet Med 32:1404–1414
19. Daniels R, van Rossum E, de Witte L et al (2008) Interventions to prevent disability in frail community-dwelling elderly: a systematic review. BMC Health Serv Res 8:278
20. Daniels R, van Rossum E, Metzelthin S et al (2011) A disability prevention programme for community-dwelling frail older persons. Clin Rehabil 25:963–974
21. Clegg A, Young J, Iliffe S, Rikkert MO et al (2013) Frailty in elderly people. Lancet 381:752–762
22. Murtagh EM, Murphy MH, Boone-Heinonen J (2010) Walking: the first steps in cardiovascular disease prevention. Curr Opin Cardiol 25:490–496
23. Edwards M, Dennison E, Sayer AA et al (2015) Osteoporosis and sarcopenia in older age. Bone 80:126–130
24. Giangregorio L, McGill S, Wark J et al (2014) Too fit to fracture: outcomes of a Delphi consensus process on physical activity and exercise recommendations for adults with osteoporosis with or without vertebral fractures. Osteoporos Int 25:821–835
25. Wendel-Vos GC, Schuit AJ, Tijhuis MA et al (2004) Leisure time physical activity and health-related quality of life: cross-sectional and longitudinal associations. Qual Life Res 13: 667–677
26. American College of Sports Medicine, Chodzko-Zajko WJ, Proctor DN, Fiatarone Singh MA et al (2009) American College of Sports Medicine position stand. Exercise and physical activity for older adults. Med Sci Sports Exerc 41:1510–1530
27. Paterson DH, Warburton DE (2010) Physical activity and functional limitations in older adults: a systematic review related to Canada's physical activity guidelines. Int J Behav Nutr Phys Act 7:38
28. Levine ME, Suarez JA, Brandhorst S et al (2014) Low protein intake is associated with a major reduction in IGF-1, cancer, and overall mortality in the 65 and younger but not older population. Cell Metab 19:407–417
29. Patterson L (2014) Making our health and care systems fit for an ageing population: David Oliver, Catherine Foot, Richard Humphries. King's Fund March 2014. Age Ageing 43:731
30. Wagner EH (2000) The role of patient care teams in chronic disease management. BMJ 320:569–572
31. Beard JR, Bloom DE (2015) Towards a comprehensive public health response to population ageing. Lancet 385:658–661
32. WHO (2007) Age-friendly cities: a guide. World Health Organization, Geneva
33. Huss A, Stuck AE, Rubenstein LZ et al (2008) Multidimensional preventive home visit programs for community-dwelling older adults: a systematic review and meta-analysis of randomized controlled trials. J Gerontol A Biol Sci Med Sci 63:298–307
34. Beswick AD, Rees K, Dieppe P et al (2008) Complex interventions to improve physical function and maintain independent living in elderly people: a systematic review and meta-analysis. Lancet 371:725–735
34. Shepperd S, Wee B, Straus SE (2011) Hospital at home: home-based end of life care. Cochrane Database Syst Rev 7:CD009231
35. Caplan GA, Sulaiman NS, Mangin DA et al (2012) A meta-analysis of "hospital in the home". Med J Aust 197:512–519

Conclusion: Moving Beyond Disease-Based Models of Prevention

20

John R. Beard

In the 2015 *World report on ageing and health,* the World Health Organization emphasised the need to consider *Healthy Ageing* from the perspective of people's functional ability to be, and to do, the things they value. This ability is determined by the intrinsic capacity of the individual (i.e. all of the individual's physical and mental, including psychosocial, capacities), the environments they inhabit, and the interaction between the individual and their environment. Furthermore, the report emphasised the importance of considering patterns of ability and capacity across people's lives.

This reframing of *Healthy Ageing* away from a conceptualisation defined by the absence of disease and towards a focus on an individual's functioning has many implications for clinicians and researchers. One of the most fundamental is a shift to considering *Healthy Ageing* as a trajectory of functioning that builds and declines across an individual's life. Interventions to promote health in older age can therefore occur at any stage of the life course, rather than being solely the domain of geriatricians. One greatly neglected area in this regard has been midlife.

While every individual's *Healthy Ageing* trajectories are unique, at a population level, people in the second half of life tend to fall into one of three groups: those with high and stable capacity, those with declining capacity and those with significant losses. The needs of each of these groups are quite distinct. Moreover, chronological age is only loosely associated with the group into which an individual falls.

The group with high and stable capacity are generally well served by existing health services, at least in high resource settings. This is a group in whom disease prevention is important and who should be encouraged and supported to avoid traditional cardiovascular risk behaviours such as smoking, lack of physical activity and poor nutrition. It is also a group where it is important to identify diseases, or risk factors such as hypertension, early and if possible cure or control them.

J. R. Beard
Department of Ageing and Life Course, World Health Organization, Geneva, Switzerland
e-mail: beardj@who.int

J.-P. Michel (ed.), *Prevention of Chronic Diseases and Age-Related Disability*, Practical Issues in Geriatrics, https://doi.org/10.1007/978-3-319-96529-1_20

At the other end of the spectrum, the group with significant losses of capacity are traditionally the domain of geriatrics and, while this area receives inadequate investment, it is a field where we generally have a good understanding of what needs to be done—typically the provision of comprehensive and integrated care that spans both health and social care services.

However, the middle group who are experiencing declines in capacity have quite different needs again, and rarely have access to the services they require. Nor do we yet have a clear understanding of the optimal interventions that might be most appropriate for them. These declines of capacity can arise from the complex multimorbidities that the majority of people over the age of 65 years experience, or they may simply reflect complex shifts in systems biology that are the consequence of diverse factors such as the accumulation of physiologic deficits across the life course or early life infections that can set in place a cascade of immune senescence and inflammageing.

Regardless of the cause, this period of many people's lives presents a significant opportunity to influence their subsequent trajectories of capacity and ability. For this is a group in whom prevention is still important, but this is not so much the prevention of disease, but rather the prevention of the declines that can be a consequence of disease and other physiologic changes. This book has explored some of these issues.

Making the most of these opportunities will require a significant shift in our thinking. For example, most current advice on physical activity emphasises the need for aerobic exercise as a preventive behaviour to reduce the risk of cardiovascular disease. Yet as declines in capacity progress, there is strong evidence that resistance training to improve muscle strength increases in importance. And there is also growing evidence that short burst high intensity training may be particularly beneficial in preventing age-related declines, at least at a cellular level. Tailoring this advice to an individual's physiologic state may be important, as is identifying the interventions and environmental context that can best encourage these activities.

Broader social advances are also creating new opportunities. For example, the advent of wearable devices means that many aspects of capacity and ability can be continuously monitored, although neither clinicians nor researchers typically make the most of the mega data that is already available. Nor do we yet have information systems that each of us might access as informed individuals to guide our personal choices and behaviours. Moreover, outdated stereotypes often cloud our thinking and can lead us to reject, or discourage in others, the activities (for example high intensity training in older adults) that might be in their best interest.

This book therefore represents an important watershed that signifies a shift from disease dominated thinking to models where diseases are still understood to be important, but are seen as both a manifestation and a contributor to complex systems that tend to decline in the second half of life. Moreover, by considering these changes in capacity within the context of an individual's physical and social environment, it highlights further opportunities to change the way we think, feel and act about ageing and to create supportive environments that can help us build and maintain capacity or compensate for losses.

While it is only a start along this path, hopefully it will encourage more research on the subtle changes that occur in midlife, and the interventions that may have the most beneficial impacts on people's subsequent lives. Then, of course, we will need to redesign our health systems and communities to draw on this knowledge to support everyone to live the longest and healthiest life possible. And in doing that, we will need to pay particular attention to those at the bottom of the range of capacity and ability who are likely to have experienced the cumulative impact of disadvantage across their lives. This is a radical transformation. However, it is one that is within our reach if we just dare to grasp the opportunity.

FSC
www.fsc.org
MIX
Papier aus verantwortungsvollen Quellen
Paper from responsible sources
FSC® C105338

If you have any concerns about our products,
you can contact us on
ProductSafety@springernature.com

In case Publisher is established outside the EU,
the EU authorized representative is:
Springer Nature Customer Service Center GmbH
Europaplatz 3, 69115 Heidelberg, Germany

Printed by Libri Plureos GmbH
in Hamburg, Germany